Praise for

AMERICAN SIRENS

"Journalist and former paramedic Kevin Hazzard paints a vivid picture of the nation's first EMS service.... His book succeeds in recalling long-overlooked events. It's a medical and human drama that will make readers appreciate the courage of the first paramedics, the foresight of a physician not content to restrict emergency medicine to other doctors, and the artistry of modern EMS workers. It's also a narrative bristling with the indignities of racism and medical ignorance. Hazzard's subjects defied and overcame prejudice but also were often overwhelmed by both.... *American Sirens* isn't a book you're likely to forget."

—*Washington Post*

"A gripping story of the people, places, and times that led to the development of Freedom House Ambulance Service, a Pittsburgh-based group of Black men whose efforts laid the foundation for the emergency medical services we take for granted today. Like many chapters of Black history, *American Sirens* is equal parts tragic and inspiring."

—Damon Tweedy, M.D., *New York Times* bestselling author of *Black Man in a White Coat: A Doctor's Reflections on Race and Medicine*

"Remarkable... there are a lot of terrific stories and interesting characters, and it's worth getting this."

—Dave Davies, "Fresh Air" (NPR)

"A riveting portrait... a fascinating and deeply rewarding study of triumph in the face of adversity." —*Publishers Weekly* (starred review)

"A work that a reads like a novel. Hazzard relates how a group of African American visionaries, most of whom had been trapped in menial jobs, saw what health-policy experts did not... After their new discipline proved its value in saving lives, organized emergency care, like so many arenas in US medicine, excluded the Black men who invented it and effaced the history of what all Americans owe them, but this riveting page-turner brings these medical heroes long-delayed acclaim."

—Harriet Washington, NBCC award–winning author of *Medical Apartheid: The Dark History of Medical Experimentation on Black Americans from Colonial Times to the Present*

"Kevin Hazzard... does an excellent job of transforming his research into a compelling narrative suitable to his gripping subject.... *American Sirens* is a stirring, ultimately heartbreaking story in which jaw-dropping medical innovation meets racial prejudice. After finishing Hazzard's memorable account, readers will never hear an ambulance siren the same way again."

—*BookPage*

"In a quintessentially American story that reads like a novel, Kevin Hazzard crafts an amazing story of an Austrian immigrant, an unlikely group of Black men, and a minority community in Pittsburgh who transformed paramedic and ambulance care throughout the United States.... This heart-warming story is not just Black history, but American history, and every American truly owes the medics of Freedom House a debt of gratitude."

—Gretchen Sorin, author of *Driving While Black: African American Travel and the Road to Civil Rights*

"Kevin Hazzard's revelatory *American Sirens* is a rich, vibrant, and deeply human look into the wild journey of American innovation. Hazzard's exacting and expansive research is deeply present on every page, yet it feels invisible, as this electric story pulses, engages, and surprises like a great novel. Each chapter unlocks a new and important angle of this almost forgotten story, which makes it almost pathologically compelling to read. *American Sirens* brings a necessary spotlight to a fascinating, near-forgotten, and uniquely American tale."

—Cristin O'Keefe Aptowicz, *New York Times* bestselling author of *Dr. Mütter's Marvels: A True Tale of Intrigue and Innovation at the Dawn of Modern Medicine*

"An amazing book: a forgotten story about real life health-care heroes inseparable from the ongoing tragedy of racism in America. Kevin Hazzard has performed a national service by writing *American Sirens*."

—Theresa Brown, RN, *New York Times* bestselling author of *The Shift: One Nurse, Twelve Hours, Four Patients' Lives*

"In this brilliant narrative, Kevin Hazzard leads us on a tour through the history of jazz, baseball, and the misnamed 'urban renewal,' to set the stage for Freedom House, a Pittsburgh ambulance service staffed by Black men, that birthed the emergency medical services we all rely on today."

—Julie Holland, MD, bestselling author of *Weekends at Bellevue: Nine Years on the Night Shift at the Psych ER*

"Hazzard has a novelist's sense of character and narrative drive. He's at his best telling the story of John Moon [which] makes for gripping and inspiring reading. And Hazzard's own experience as a paramedic helps us understand why achievements like Moon's learning how to do an intubation in the field was such a big deal.... Readers of *American Sirens* will be more than satisfied, and can hope Hazzard has helped revive and secure the legacy of everyone who breathed Freedom House into life."

—*Pittsburgh Post-Gazette*

"If readers have ever wondered about the history of paramedicine and how it can transform lives (paramedic and patient alike), look no further than this wonderful, enlightening work by former paramedic [Kevin] Hazzard. . . . Through extensive research and interviews, the author successfully incorporates the checkered history of paramedicine with the racial and social history of the mid-twentieth century. Furthermore, he engages the reader with the personal stories of all those involved in the development of the new system. Hazzard has fashioned an exceptional work about radical changes in health care and the importance of community in dark times."

—*Library Journal*

AMERICAN SIRENS

Also by Kevin Hazzard

A Thousand Naked Strangers: A Paramedic's Wild Ride to the Edge and Back

AMERICAN SIRENS

THE INCREDIBLE STORY OF THE BLACK MEN WHO BECAME AMERICA'S FIRST PARAMEDICS

KEVIN HAZZARD

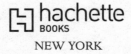

NEW YORK

Cover design by Terri Sirma
Cover photograph: image from The National EMS Museum Photograph Collection; texture © IgorGolovniov/Shutterstock

Hachette Books
Hachette Book Group
1290 Avenue of the Americas
New York, NY 10104
HachetteBooks.com
Twitter.com/HachetteBooks
Instagram.com/HachetteBooks

First Trade Paperback Edition: January 2024

Published by Hachette Books, an imprint of Perseus Books, LLC, a subsidiary of Hachette Book Group, Inc. The Hachette Books name and logo is a trademark of the Hachette Book Group.

Print book interior design by Linda Mark

Library of Congress Cataloging-in-Publication Data
Names: Hazzard, Kevin M., 1977– author.
Title: American sirens : the incredible story of the Black men who became America's first paramedics / Kevin Hazzard.
Description: First edition. | New York : Hachette Books, 2022. | Includes bibliographical references.
Identifiers: LCCN 2022006917 | ISBN 9780306926075 (hardcover) | ISBN 9780306926082 (ebook)
Subjects: LCSH: Freedom House Ambulance Service (Pittsburgh, Pa.) | Emergency medical technicians—Pennsylvania—Pittsburgh—Biography | Ambulance service—Pennsylvania—Pittsburgh—History—20th century.
Classification: LCC RA645.6.P4 H39 2022 | DDC 362.18/809748/86—dc23/eng/20220609
LC record available at https://lccn.loc.gov/2022006917

ISBNs: 9780306926075 (hardcover), 9780306926099 (trade paperback), 9780306926082 (ebook)

Printed in the United States of America

LSC-C

Printing 1, 2023

For Pepe, as always

and

To John, who continues to answer the call

The revolution will not be televised.

—Gil Scott-Heron

CONTENTS

AMERICAN SIRENS

PROLOGUE

It took Ragin screaming in their faces on the corner of Fifth and Market for people to notice him. That's how easy he was to ignore. Thin, light-skinned, glasses. And those clothes, you know the clothes, almost a uniform for people living on the streets—dirty jeans and too-large shoes, shirt upon shirt upon shirt. The sort of guy people ignore until he's shouting at them, and then it's like he appeared from nowhere, by magic, a problem without a source, angry and raising hell over crimes committed against him yesterday or the week before, maybe a decade before. But he kept turning it up and eventually got so combative someone called the cops, which says something about how worked up he was, considering, in the early '80s, Pittsburgh's Market Square was overrun by crime and drugs, by pigeons. By countless men just like this one. People did their best to keep moving, one look—*don't look*—and you're sucked in. Now they were sucked in, all those people staring. And not one of them knew his name.

Across town, John Moon sat in a four-wheel-drive Suburban with his job (Pittsburgh EMS) and title (supervisor) painted on the door. Outwardly John seemed constructed to blend, with his average height and weight, those soft features. Inside he was a bundle of contrasts. Northern raised but a Southern accent. Mid-thirties but a string of past lives. Loved Angela Davis and the afro but polite to the point (almost) of deference. He wore silver-framed glasses that he occasionally slid back into place with a long, thin finger. Inside his car, the radio played softly, a Jackie Wilson song maybe or the jazz guitar of Wes Montgomery. His truck was spotless, gleaming, the uniform freshly pressed. Everything about him, all that he owned, was carefully tended with the meticulous pride of a man who once had nothing. Outside his window, clouds slipped past in the Pittsburgh sky.

Back at Market Square, the police arrived with a slam of car doors. Ragin was wound up, and they watched from a distance, sifting through a thousand scenarios for the one that brought this . . . whatever you wanted to call it, to an end the quickest. Contain and control. One of the cops reached for his radio.

The two-way in John's truck crackled. Along with radio traffic from his crews on the street, he kept an ear on the police radio too. Better to know what's coming before it arrives. What arrived that afternoon, floating up from the speaker in a burst of static, caught his attention: "Black male at Fifth and Market. Possible psych. Combative." John knew without having to be told that it was Ragin in the street. That he could get angry and loud and that when he did, people got nervous. He knew that Ragin had peered over the edge and slipped, that he'd come untethered from reality and probably he was harmless, but the cops didn't know that, and they were in charge now. What they did next could be anything. John slipped the key into the ignition, turned it, and pumped the gas pedal until the Suburban roared to life.

Downtown Pittsburgh is a near-perfect triangle of land formed by the Monongahela and Allegheny rivers as they join to create a third, the Ohio, a confluence marked by the site of the eighteen-century remains of Fort Duquesne—a trophy from the French and Indian War known now as Point State Park. A few blocks to the east sits Market Square, and it's here, next to an oyster house that was once (maybe) a stop along the Underground Railroad, that John found Ragin wrestling with the cops.

John cursed out loud, then yanked the wheel and pulled the Suburban to a quick stop along the curb, reaching for the two-way radio to tell the dispatcher he was on-scene.

"Medic 30." Already throwing the truck into park.

"Go ahead, Medic 30," the dispatcher called back.

"Show me out at Fifth and Market." Swinging open the door.

Market Square tingled with the electric pulse of danger. The crowd was jittery and tense as Ragin—scared, angry, and disoriented, rapidly coming unspooled in the street—screamed at the cops, who in turn had a hold of his arms and were trying to drag him to the ground. The cops hadn't yet hit him or cuffed him, but John could feel their anger and frustration even from here, on the outer edges of the crowd. He stepped into the clearing.

"Mind if I try?"

One of the cops swung his head just enough to catch the white gleam of a uniform as John, hands on hips, drew to a stop with the deliberate assurance of a conductor appraising his audience. This nonchalance was a learned habit, the product of over a dozen years on an ambulance, leaping daily onto the back of emergencies big and small. To practice medicine in the street a paramedic must first gain control of the environment—come in too hot, swept up in the panic and rush, and everything goes to hell. Instead, John approached Ragin and the cops, too, the way he would any scene. Like a drop of reason in the swirling waters of chaos. He nodded toward Ragin.

"I know him. Why don't you let me have a word?" John's voice was gentle, half an octave higher than you'd expect, a syrupy Southern accent kids had once mocked him for smoothed over by time to a rolling lilt. He now had both cops' attention and kept talking, asking how and when all this started, and after a moment—John standing there the whole time, an easy presence within arm's reach—they let go of Ragin. With the fighting stopped, the screaming stopped too. Tension broke all at once like a release valve had finally burst open, and at last everyone could breathe.

John stepped forward, the crowd still watching. He kept his hands relaxed at his sides, his voice just loud enough to be heard.

"How's it going, Ragin?" Nothing. "What's going on?"

John kept at it, easing close but not too close, trying to penetrate the fog of psychosis or alcohol or drugs—or maybe all three—not to mention the fear and anger, the confusion of the moment. When he got within whispering distance, Ragin finally turned to him, his face twisted and angry, eyes vacant. John pressed on.

"It's John." A smile. "Remember?"

A look of recognition flashed in Ragin's eyes, though it might've been only the recognition that John's was a friendly face. He relaxed as the coiled spring inside him slowly went loose. That was the signal the cops had been waiting for, the evidence of de-escalation that freed them from having to fix the situation, and they slowly returned to their car with an air of nothing-to-see-here that rippled through the crowd.

As everyone left, John ushered Ragin to a low stone wall, where the two men leaned in silence while Ragin caught his breath. These two had once known each other, in a different time, another life, but to look at the man before him now made John's heart sink. This wasn't Ragin, not really. John had bumped into him here recently, on a good day, when Ragin knew who and where he was, yet even then John could see the issues. Covered over but not hidden, exacerbated by alcohol and drugs.

What set him off this afternoon John couldn't say, though how the two of them ended up here, at Market Square, one wearing a supervisor's uniform, the other a moldering bundle of clothes, was a story neither new nor unique whose details, like songlines, reached back over decades and across borders to trace the geography of their lives. It started just a few blocks from where they now stood, in the basement of Presbyterian-University Hospital, when a small group of Black men—some forty-four students in all—were selected to take the world's first paramedic course. Nothing of its kind, not even the word *paramedic*, existed at the time, and yet they dedicated themselves to it, paused and even walked away from their lives for it. Nearly a year of intense study followed, a long swim in water so deep that half of them, submerged to near-drowning, didn't finish. Those who did would go on to staff a pioneering ambulance service called Freedom House, work that would change the world, truly, and inspire a whole nation—John included—to follow them. Ragin had been one of those men.

He'd been part of a new era in emergency medicine, took ideas, practices, and technology just then being developed and carried it all out into the street to serve a population who for decades had little access to health care and even less reason to believe that, when it finally arrived, it would be delivered by their own neighbors. He was part of the front line, forever changing how Americans live and die.

That Ragin and the rest of the original class were Black men would've been remarkable now, in 1984, or even a decade earlier, but in '67, when they started, it was unthinkable. They got pushback from all sides, hand-wringing and head-shaking that carried with it the usual justifications, but the subtext was there, it'd always been there, and sometimes it wasn't even subtext, but the *actual* text. Even as Freedom House was making history, across town a white truck driver passing a line of Black demonstrators protesting discriminatory hiring practices in the construction industry leaned from the window of his truck to yell, "Want a job, n—s? Join the army!" It was the same old story, the anger of one part of America brought to bear against the wishes of another. The paramedics knew it well.

As much as possible they ignored it—the job was too consuming, too important—but still it felt as if the whole thing was built to fail. Probably that's what made the way it ended so painful. They didn't fail. They succeeded, wildly. Paramedicine as they practiced it—practically invented it—worked; it saved lives. It became a fixture, spawned a subculture, inspired a hit TV show. It was the rare innovation so intuitive and obvious that in hindsight no one could imagine or even remember a life without it. But in the end that wasn't enough, and the Freedom House medics were replaced by people who followed what they did but looked nothing like them at all.

The way it ended affected each of the guys who'd been there differently. Some went on to other fields, other cities. For Ragin, maybe the best paramedic of them all, it meant a slow tumble from normal life. Underemployment, then unemployment, living on one or another of his friends' couches until he ran out of couches. Out of friends. And now he was here.

Things had gone differently for John. Asked how he had defied the odds to survive and keep climbing, John would point to an unstable life made harder by fate. He started with nothing then lost even that, but he refused to go away. And it was in the fighting back that he found reserves of strength and a fierce self-reliance fueled by a wild anger that roiled just beneath the surface.

The same forces that tried to bury him—redlining, urban renewal, poverty, indifference, racism—had ultimately turned him into a survivor, and in that sense, though John wasn't the first or the best, he perfectly embodied all that Freedom House had stood for.

And now here he stood, next to a man whose fate by almost any measure should've been his own. Maybe Ragin was Freedom House, too, just one more facet of a proud but complicated legacy. John turned to him, nodded.

"Ragin, man, how you doing?"

A lot had changed since those days. And a lot hadn't, so much that it made you wonder if things would ever change.

"It's John." He held a fist out for Ragin to thump. "From Freedom House. I know you remember that."

BOOK ONE

CHAPTER ONE

On a night like any other, pinned somewhere along the dreary timeline of another cold, endless Pittsburgh winter, two men entered Montefiore Hospital and changed the trajectory of John Moon's life.

It was 1971, the year of the Pentagon Papers and the Attica Prison Riot, the year Disney World opened and Jim Morrison died. John was twenty-two, on his own, and working his second job since graduating high school. His first didn't last long. The J&L Steel Mill was a tough place, dangerous and exhausting, barely worth the effort—what good was money you were too tired to enjoy? Not that he could just up and quit. He had a wife, Betty, whom he'd met in high school. They married in 1969, and their first son, John Jr., was born later that year. Even with Betty working as a nurse's aide at Shadyside Hospital, money was tight. If John was going to quit, he'd need something else first. One day at work he was talking about wanting to get out of the steel mill, his friends just nodding along, when one of them made a suggestion. He knew of a job, he said. Good money, no two days the same, career field with a thousand options. Sky's the limit. John asked what it was, and the guy pointed at him as if he'd laid his finger on the truth and said, "Hospital orderly."

By '71, John had been listening to the *sploosh* of bedpans emptying for almost three years, feeling that somewhere along the way he'd taken a wrong turn, that there had to be something more. And then, as he stuffed a set of rumpled sheets into a hamper, that something more walked into his life.

It was late when it happened. John was working in Two East, one of Montefiore's oldest wings—now full of cancer patients, surgical cases—when from the far end of a quiet and otherwise deserted corridor he heard garbled voices coming in over a two-way radio. He'd just stepped into a patient's room and couldn't see where the sound was coming from until it passed right by the door. Two figures, large and moving slowly, draped head to toe in white like angels from a high school passion play. John thought they might be orderlies too, but why they'd be here on his floor, with a radio, he couldn't imagine.

"I'll be right back," he whispered to his patient before stepping outside to get a better look.

He got only as far as the doorway when the stretcher came jamming into the room, John barely out of the way in time to keep from being run over by two men in white and the charge nurse right behind them. Nobody so much as glanced in his direction, as if he wasn't there at all. One minute John's taking care of a patient, the next minute the patient is theirs.

"Mr. Smith," the first man said as he eased up alongside the bed. "We're here to take you home."

The patient looked up with the placid, animal eyes of a man with no control over the moment. "Is it cold?"

"Sure is," said the second man as he slid their stretcher alongside the bed. "But we got a blanket here for you, so you're gonna be just fine."

One, two, go, and they lifted the patient, swiftly, with great care, onto their stretcher, then buckled the lap belt with a sharp *click*. John still had no idea who these guys were except to say that they definitely weren't orderlies. Their uniforms were white like his but cut differently—more like button-up jackets with Nehru collars and sewn-on patches—plus there was the radio that one of them wore on his hip.

John couldn't take his eyes off the radio. It was turned down to a whisper but never silent, filling the air with a stream of encoded words he didn't understand, like distant voices reaching out from some other planet. Now with the patient loaded, they were leaving. Once again they eased right by John and slipped out with a nod to the nurse. Here was a woman who only ever acknowledged John when she needed something, a patient needing to be moved or those damn bedpans, but he couldn't help but notice that now, to these guys, she nodded back.

The men moved back down the hall as if gliding, silent except for the alien murmur of the two-way, then rounded a corner, and with that they were gone. The whole encounter hadn't taken thirty seconds.

John looked around the empty room, wondering if he'd really seen what he'd just seen or if it was all in his head, one of those tricks the mind plays in the quiet hallucinatory hours at the end of a long night shift. His thoughts spun and whirred, questions, ideas, realizations, but all he managed to say—and he said it out loud, astonished and in disbelief—was, "Those were *Black* guys."

There's no way to overstate this, the *rarity*, in 1971, for a pair of Black men to wander into a hospital as if they owned the place, autonomous of its hierarchy, in a role they alone occupied and controlled. They carried themselves confidently and boldly, as if they not only belonged but were in charge. John looked around. "How are they able to do *that*?"

Before he even realized what he was doing, John was out the door and halfway down the hall. He was supposed to be stripping sheets from the bed, cleaning the room for whatever patient came next, or prepping another for discharge or surgery, some menial orderly task. Instead, he slipped around the corner and reached the elevator in a near trot and pressed the down arrow, waited impatiently for the car to arrive, then stepped inside and madly pressed the button for the ground floor.

The doors shuddered open, and John rushed out into the quiet of an empty hall. No sign of the men or their patient or the radio. He tried to guess which way they'd gone but couldn't be certain. Montefiore was originally built in 1929, had been expanding ever since, and was now less a hospital than a constellation of buildings spread over entire city blocks.

There was no telling where they were. They were gone.

WHY JOHN WAS in the hospital that night had as much to do with the mundane realities of scheduling as it did with pure, unforeseen chance.

Life as an orderly wasn't inspiring, but it was steady and honest and wouldn't have been that bad—as far as first(ish) jobs go—if it hadn't been for the fact that every day the important work of saving lives was happening all around him. Initially built to serve the city's Jewish population, Montefiore had joined the ranks of research and teaching facilities in 1957, when it became part of the University of Pittsburgh's medical system. By the time John arrived a little over a decade later, he was surrounded by technology and equipment, an assembly of minds and ideas that brought the full power of Western medicine to bear in the battle to preserve human life. That spirit of wonder and excitement, that glamour, was in the air, and it buoyed everyone around him. The doctors were young and perched atop a pedestal; when not treating patients, they were chasing the nurses who seemed dead set on marrying a doctor, which made them easy, almost jubilant prey.

For the orderlies, almost all of whom were Black, it was different. John was at the bottom of the ladder or near to it at least. One step up from the janitors, depending on who was asking. Orderlies were a necessary evil, something to be tolerated and utilized but never engaged or included. Unless something went missing from a patient's room, and then the first glance of suspicion was always cast at the orderlies. *They're known for stealing things, you know.* In good times when things were running as they should, and the floor wasn't understaffed or overcrowded, when a patient's watch and rings, her necklaces, billfold, and silk scarf all sat untouched and accounted for at the foot of her bed, no one wanted to talk to the orderlies. The patients took note of this and, along with whatever suppositions they'd carried in with them, treated John—even as they looked to him for comfort and compassion—much as the doctors and nurses did. And the doctors and nurses treated him as if they existed on another plane. In many ways, they did.

Working for, around, and beneath doctors, handling the messy, menial jobs that no one else would touch, John wondered why he couldn't do more. It was the same vague notion of wanting to be bigger and more important, to be better, that had made him restless at the steel mill, only here, at Montefiore, his drive crystallized into a clear-eyed goal. Inside these walls, John could be more than just a scared child or an angry teenager, a frustrated young man trying to provide for a family. Limited as it was, the job revealed a potential for compassion and empathy that he didn't know he possessed and that could, if allowed to grow, give him an identity. Medicine was the place where he could make his mark, but how he'd take that next step and begin this journey wasn't at all clear. Until now.

And so alone in the hospital's predawn quiet, he was kicking himself. All that night and into the next morning, he couldn't shake the feeling that somewhere out there guys very much like him were getting to do something he'd never imagined possible, and that their arrival had presented an opportunity—or at least its possibility—but he'd let it slip away.

Two weeks later, John was in the OR, sent to roll a patient from surgery back to the wing. He didn't know that a mile away, maybe less, maybe within walking distance, as he unlocked the stretcher to begin his trek to Two East, an emergency was happening. They happen all the time, disasters unfolding in a minor key, too small to be noticed by anyone but those sent in to fix them. It could've been anything, but probably the whole thing unfolded like this.

It starts with a phone call. There's no preamble for rescuers. One minute they're laughing or reading, finally set to take the first bite of a sandwich they've waited all night to eat, and then the phone rings.

The dispatcher answers, and the two men next up freeze, motionless except for their eyes, which cut from each other to her and back. Waiting for the sign, hopping up when they get it. The details of the call are quickly jotted down on a piece of paper ripped from a pad and handed over as they hustle out. A million things separate doctors from medics, and among them, on a list that includes education and training and pay, overlooked by everyone who's never confronted the peculiar realities of the job, is that medics have no specialty. They're expected to handle anything from a human in labor to a human on fire. Often consecutively and in no particular order. The call that night in Pittsburgh could've been an assault at the Bedford Dwellings, an overdose on Crawford, or a shooting in Homewood. Maybe a jumper on the Fort Duquesne Bridge. Or the Fort Pitt Bridge. Or any of the bridges spanning Sixth, Seventh, Ninth, or Tenth streets.

But probably it's a middle-aged man with chest pain and difficulty breathing. It is most certainly on a street they know well and walked as boys, a home they've passed a thousand times. It's entirely possible that whoever's dying that night is someone they know. Once they pull up in their ambulance, they rush in and set to work immediately. There's so little time when someone's slipping through your fingers. Maybe family members are screaming from the edge of that chaotic little bubble as the paramedics lay their patient flat on the floor and open his shirt.

A quick check for breathing—nope—then a breath of stale air from a portable device called a bag-valve mask. Then another. Fill the lungs. Next a pulse check—nope again. Their own pulses by now are bounding. The patient will be lost soon, beyond reach, and that realization, the adrenaline, it's overwhelming.

They begin CPR right there on the floor. Two hands placed over the breastbone for fifteen compressions followed by two breaths, a cycle they repeat without pause all the way to the hospital. But first they've got to carry him down the steps and across the lawn, bundle him into the ambulance for the mad rush across the city. When they get to Montefiore, the driver hops out and helps his partner with the stretcher, and together they rush their dying patient through the doors, banging from darkness into light.

And John just so happened to be standing there when they did.

He'd dropped his patient off on Two East and was on break and near the entrance when the quiet of a late-night hospital was interrupted by a burst of chaos. The doors flung open, and there they were, the guys he'd seen before. Maybe not the same guys, but from the same place. That much he knew. He recognized the jackets. And their attitude. But this time there was no ease to their step, no gentle murmur from the radio. They were all intensity, working desperately on the lifeless patient flopped on their stretcher, hauling ass, and headed right for him.

John jumped out of the way. He pressed his back to the wall, and everything began to slow. His eyes fell to the patient, limp and half-covered beneath a single sheet. He looked to the guys pushing the stretcher. One held the portable ventilator to the patient's face with his bare hands, breathing for him with each careful squeeze of the bag. He was focused and alert, attuned, fully in rhythm with the patient's dire state. His partner on the other side of the stretcher wasn't looking at the patient at all but rather somewhere down the hall. John followed his gaze and saw a doctor. The man beckoned to the physician with a single outstretched arm, and without hesitation the doctor followed them around the corner and into a room.

And just that fast they were gone. The quiet of night returned as if nothing had ever happened. Swallowed them right up. John stood with his back pressed to the cold tile wall, thinking about what he'd just seen. Their white jackets carried words that were opaque to him. On a round patch, the words *Freedom House Ambulance* formed a circle around a medical cross. Stitched on their breast pockets was *paramedic*.

Five minutes ago, the word would've meant nothing, but now. . . . In John's mind it summed up their ability and focus, the hardened look of confidence in their eyes. The fact that a doctor had followed them, taken orders from them. The word was a mystery, an answer to a question he didn't know how to ask.

Somewhere out there, beyond the doors of the hospital, something important was happening, something that couldn't be ignored. Through his quiet years and then the angry ones when he was unreachable and out of control, the extravagant ones, too, when he walked down the street in the loudest clothes he could find—*all eyes on me*—that whole time what John wanted was a place in this world where he felt he counted. For years his life was something that happened to him, as if he was there but not essential. Helplessness. Frustration. Anger. It all stemmed from a nagging sense of insignificance, but here, packed inside this word—*paramedic*—was a way to be seen. To matter.

CHAPTER TWO

John Moon was born in Atlanta, at Grady Memorial, a hospital that hid his mother away in its Black-only section like a secret so that none of its staff or equipment, not even the bed onto which he was delivered, would be used for white babies. The city was and remains ambivalent about this legacy. Grady's an Atlanta institution, loved and hated, vitally necessary and yet was so strictly segregated that even after its 1965 integration it was still referred to as the Gradies. It has always sat in the historic heart of Black Atlanta, Sweet Auburn, just a few doors down from the spot where Alonzo Herndon, formerly enslaved, opened the Atlanta Life Insurance Company and became the city's first Black millionaire. Grady is also the place where, just four months after John was born, *Gone with the Wind* author Margaret Mitchell died after being struck by a car on Peachtree Street. It is an auspicious place to begin life.

John began his on April 2, 1949, the first of two children for Elzora and Clinton Moon. By the time his sister, June, was born two years later, the family lived just north of downtown in a tangle of unpaved side streets and alleyways known as Buttermilk Bottom. How to describe the Bottom? It was a mid-twentieth-century urban neighborhood banished, by decree and neglect, to a nineteenth-century existence, named for the smell of sewage backflowing into the street, and whose two thousand residents, African Americans mostly, worked as help in the nearby mansions. By the time John came along, most of those big houses were gone, victims either to fire or progress, and so jobs, like electricity and phone or trash service, were something people in Buttermilk Bottom didn't have. Occasionally, because they could, drunk white men drove through at night firing guns.

The Moons lived on Ellis Street, the southern fringe of the neighborhood, in a tiny house with a tar-paper roof, a wood-burning stove, kerosene lamps, and no indoor plumbing. Wedged alongside them and heading off in every direction were cobbled-together shacks with boards missing from the walls. In some places the shacks had been replaced by decrepit two-story apartments with sagging porches that swayed under the weight of children at play. Stilts and cinder blocks lifted homes above the trash and standing water that lined the streets, and that helped but not enough. Typhoid remained an occasional but stubborn problem.

The Moonses' house had a single room and one bed the whole family slept in. A log had to be lit to cook even the simplest of meals, though there wasn't much to cook anyhow. The children went without food and shoes, without going to school. John and June had no idea they were poor, and Clinton, who worked as a handyman, was gone all day. So it was Elzora, stuck at home with no distractions, no wonderful and youthful ignorance of what was happening, who suffered the most. She understood perfectly well where she was and that she'd never get out, a permanence she never seemed to square with. Her truth tomorrow was her truth today, a life in which every drop of water had to be carted in from outside, in which needs were ignored because they couldn't be met. Her life was a trap to be escaped. So she drank.

"Long as I'm not working," she'd say, "I can get drunk."

Alcohol was a way of life in the Bottom, most of it moonshine. A couple times a week bootleggers disappeared, off to some hidden still on the outskirts of town. When they returned, the trunks of their mud-spattered cars were full of moonshine, which was then hidden under the eaves of a safehouse and sold by the jar. It was public knowledge, but you drank it privately at home. Get caught drinking outside—or even inside but visible from outside—and the cops hauled you off to jail. So Elzora drank at home. Every day she'd scrape together what money she could, then head out, returning a few minutes later with a jar tucked under her arm. It was an action that became the routine, background music as John played in the yard. He'd hear the clinking of coins and a slamming door, footsteps down the front walk. The metallic *zing* of a tin lid turning loose atop a glass mason jar. It was only later, after John was grown and had watched his friends and neighbors struggle to find their own way, that he realized for his mother these were the sounds of escape, but also confinement, the whole thing a prelude to the warm splash of moonshine burning down her throat and settling in her stomach. Most nights Clinton came home to find her passed out and the kids running free. He'd wake her, and then came the fighting and yelling, the cussing, both kids slipping out of sight until it was over.

For John, staying home with a mom who was there, but also not, had its perks. He and June got their affection and attention from Clinton, so what they felt was less neglect than freedom. John woke early and got dressed. Breakfast was whatever he could scrounge, lunch too, and then he was out the door. He ran the dusty alleys, played among the heaps of scrap wood and old tires. He hung around with the other kids, threw rocks and raised hell, but his favorite spot was under the house. He'd shimmy under the porch and lie there, unseen, watching. Mostly it was just people walking by. Arguing, laughing. Living their lives.

Sometimes it was more. The cops came a lot. John would watch as they walked around looking for moonshine, jabbing their metal-tipped canes under the houses to smash the jars. It was futile; surely even the cops knew that for every mason jar they burst, plenty more made their way in. Certainly, John knew it. Heard the creak of the floorboards above his head, Elzora's footsteps down the front walk.

The *zing* of the lid. He heard it but didn't realize how much. It was too much.

It happened in October 1956. His mother went over to a neighbor's house and stayed late, drank until she passed out, and had to be carried home. Everyone in the Bottom kept their windows open to ease the stifling heat, and as the children slept, the steady thrum of cicadas from outside was suddenly replaced by muffled curses as Clinton struggled to get Elzora up the steps and into the house. John woke to the sound of boots shuffling on the bare wood floor as his mother was placed down beside him. Then the noise settled. So did John. He rolled over and drifted back to sleep. A few hours later he was up again.

"John."

It was Clinton, shaking him. "Get up. Get up, now."

John slowly opened his eyes and looked around. It was dark, and June was asleep. His mother was there too, though she hadn't moved. His father stood over him.

"Go on next door," Clinton said, an edge to his voice. "Take June with you. And you stay there till I tell you."

John rose and woke June. Together in pajamas, they tiptoed through the dirt to their neighbor's house, and there they waited, uncertain and scared. Eventually, a couple men came and removed their mother's body, but John still couldn't make sense of what was happening, too young to understand this was forever, that all those trips down the alley for mason jars had added up, each sip slowly stealing her away.

Notice of Elzora's passing was listed among the city's "colored" obituaries in the *Atlanta Constitution*, and the day after that, October 18, 1956, she was laid to rest at Hanley's Bell Street Funeral Home, the same place where, twelve years later, the Reverend Martin Luther King Jr.'s family would gather before his burial. John was lifted so he could get one last look at his mother before they closed her coffin.

He was seven years old.

What followed was hazy, confusing, the murk of clouds and a storm-tossed sea. Days, weeks, months—ultimately an entire year—passed in a blur of flattened time. Unable to fully comprehend that their mother was gone and would never return, John and June were nonetheless left to pick up the pieces and divine not just what had happened but also where to go from there. Their father was the one they'd always clung to, and while that bond remained, strengthened even, things were different. Clinton was gone most of the time when Elzora was alive, and that didn't change just because she was dead. He went to work every morning, except now John and June were left *alone*. John was expected to take care of himself and his younger sister, to not burn the house down, and also, come evening, to be there waiting when their father got home.

But home, too, became an ephemeral concept, shifting and insecure. There was talk of a highway coming through, of the government taking their land.

"Ain't no negotiating," John heard his father say. "No trying to buy the house, assistance—nothing. They're just coming."

The future was finally arriving in Buttermilk Bottom, and it most definitely would not include the people who lived there. A highway was slated to run through the center of town, and it would claim a number of homes, while a plan for urban renewal (which appeared time and again in John's life) just then being drawn up would take care of the rest.

In being evicted, having their home demolished and neighbors scattered, the Moons weren't alone. Coast to coast, Americans were being kicked loose and sent adrift by forces beyond their control. Just a few years later, in 1962, more than twenty thousand Black families would lose not only their homes but their neighborhoods and friends, all sense of community—everything—to a sweeping and ambitious but viciously destructive policy known as urban renewal. Under this program, which began in 1955 and ran into the '70s, the federal government paid for cities to tear down and then redevelop neighborhoods where housing and infrastructure were deemed substandard.

This meant that families who'd built a life amid all this substandard housing and infrastructure, quite often Black, watched as their homes were condemned and then torn down, their stores, churches, and corner hangouts all leveled. Entire streets were rerouted or simply disappeared, until finally the map of what had been was empty. They were promised, in exchange for all this, public or subsidized housing, though in the end this too proved to be empty.

But life is subjective, and to the other America, the one that would never taste the dust of its own pulverized homes, urban renewal was the chemical bond that linked exploding mid-century ambitions with edgy Cold War jitters. In the 1950s, American cities—the lifeblood of US industrial power—were belly-flopping. White Flight. The proliferation of cars. Businesses lighting out for the boonies, where land was abundant and cheap. Like any migration there was a whole raft of reasons why cities were emptying, but taken in the aggregate it meant that the suburb was now king. Urban America was rapidly drained of residents, businesses, and, most importantly, money. In New York and Chicago—not to mention the hundreds of smaller towns like San Antonio and Tacoma, which had far less cash on hand—the situation was dire. Alarmists picked up on the thread, depicting all this inner-city decay as something that the Soviet Union, which after all was out there somewhere, lurking, could prey upon. An influx of federal construction dollars to rebuild the cities and project American power seemed a perfect way to save the country from threats both within and without.

Grant applications—approved almost immediately—started rolling in, their freshly typed pages setting in motion thousands of wrecking balls that wouldn't stop swinging for nearly two decades. Whole neighborhoods were razed. In their place came highways, medical centers, and shopping malls. New York City got the Lincoln Center;

Milwaukee got a significantly expanded Marquette University; Portland expanded Legacy Emanuel Hospital.

By the early '60s, billions had been spent on urban renewal, and tens of thousands of houses were being torn down every year. Philadelphia, San Francisco, Boston, Portland—more than six hundred cities emerged from the waters born again. Urban renewal was changing the face of America with little thought given to the fate of the removed. The universities and the highways, all those shopping centers, they each cost a community its home. In Southern California, three hundred Mexican American families were evicted from Chavez Ravine to make way for what was to be a housing project but instead became a brand-new baseball stadium built as part of Los Angeles's successful bid to lure the Dodgers out of Brooklyn.

"URBAN RENEWAL . . . MEANS Negro removal." When James Baldwin said these words on May 24, 1963, he was in a state of high agitation. The intellectual, writer, and activist had just come from a meeting with Attorney General Robert Kennedy that devolved into a shouting match over race relations in Northern cities. Afterward, Baldwin was scheduled to record an interview with psychologist and activist Dr. Kenneth Clark, who'd also been present at the meeting with Kennedy. Baldwin was so flustered he tried to beg off, suggesting they go out for a drink instead. But the interview went on as scheduled, and after collecting his thoughts, Baldwin trained his fury on the truths and effects of urban renewal.

"A boy last week, he was sixteen in San Francisco, told me . . . he said, 'I got no country. I got no flag.' And I couldn't say, 'you do.' I don't have the evidence to prove that he does." In grainy black-and-white footage Baldwin weaves in his seat, bobbing as if to dodge some ugly truth buzzing around his head. "They were tearing down his house because San Francisco is engaging, as most Northern cities are now engaged, in something called urban renewal. Which means getting Negros out."

The slums slated for demolition were largely Black and had been created by the very system that now considered them a barrier to progress. The evidence was everywhere. Take redlining, in which federal and local governments, along with the private sector, actively worked together to deny entire neighborhoods home loans and essential services. The residents of these areas slated for "renewal" were minorities, underserved and overcharged, unable to improve what they owned or buy homes elsewhere. The neighborhoods became segregated became ghettos became slums, and now the slums were being torn down. With no provision for those who lived there.

The numbers are jarring.

In Philadelphia and Detroit, more than two-thirds of the families removed were minorities. In Durham, North Carolina, the number was 74 percent, while in St. Louis it was nearly 95. Almost thirteen hundred minority families in Lubbock, Texas. Five thousand in Cincinnati. The housing that was promised in exchange was delayed, was inadequate, or simply never arrived. Displaced families were crammed into communities already pressed to the edge. Overcrowding was so bad in Chicago that children had to take shifts going to school, half in the morning and half in the afternoon. Same in Cleveland. Similar stories played out in Newark, in Harlem and Watts, in Memphis, places that unsurprisingly would become flashpoints for the riots of the mid-1960s. To wit: the 1966 Hough Riots in Cleveland closely followed the relocation of a large number of Black families to Garden Valley, a housing project built on a dump.

Back in Atlanta, housing was torn down to expand Georgia Tech. The neighborhoods of Mechanicsville, Peoplestown, and Summerville were demolished to make way for Fulton County Stadium, which helped coax the Braves out of Milwaukee. And finally, after years of speculation and whispers, the wrecking ball came for Buttermilk

Bottom, where John grew up. Its three thousand people were removed and their homes demolished to build a highway and a civic center. Of all the thousands who lost their homes—residents of a modern city who for so long lived without power or running water, who stepped over sewage backflowing onto their dirt streets—only a fraction would be offered housing in the newly developed Bedford Pines housing project.

Homes gone. Communities erased. And in their wake, a profound sense of dispossession one psychiatrist called "rootshock." Nearly 98 percent of Atlantans who would experience, in one form or another, rootshock were people of color.

"Now we're talking about human beings," James Baldwin said that May afternoon in 1963, his eyes perhaps not dodging but attempting to pin down the culprit. "Not some abstraction called the Negro Problem. These are Negro boys and girls."

SPECIFICALLY, THEY WERE John and June.

When the family was put out, gone too was John's safe place beneath the eave and the bedroom he'd once shared with his mother. The Moons moved, then moved again. The rumors continued: a highway was coming through; things were being built. No one seemed to know the where or the when, just that it was happening, so they had to get out. And they did. Time and again they moved.

The stress of it wore on Clinton. He was a widower with two children and a low-paying job that mostly kept him away from home, which wasn't even home but a series of houses they fell into and then were chased out of. He couldn't keep on like that. It was rough for him and worse for his children, who were left to raise themselves, and how that would turn out, whether they'd have a chance to make something of themselves before the world swallowed them whole, he could only guess.

"GET IN THE truck."

As their father opened the door, John and June climbed in. John watched out the window as the dirt alleys of Buttermilk Bottom gave way to the paved streets of Atlanta. He stared at the high-rises springing up along Peachtree and the trains crossing the tracks that ran near Marietta Street. Then they headed down Northside Drive, skirting along the edge of an affluent African American neighborhood called Vine City. They were headed south of the city now, and John knew if they went far enough, down past the edge of town, they'd be in the land of the chain gangs, where prisoners walked like ghosts among the pines.

But they weren't going that far. Barely three and a half miles from home, Clinton eased his truck to a stop on Roy Street, a quiet little road on the south side of the city. The kids piled out of the truck and followed their father toward a building that looked to John like a store. They passed through a set of double doors, and a woman was there to greet them. She motioned for Clinton to enter the office, then turned to John and June.

"Your father's gonna talk with some people," she said, gesturing toward a playground they could see through the window. "Why don't you play outside?"

God in heaven, hallelujah. A playground, a real one, no pretending or imagining, no pile of trash, nothing cobbled together. John and June played until their father came out to say it was time to go and had so much fun that the next time the three of them piled into the truck and drove to Roy Street, they didn't hesitate when they arrived, but darted through the entryway of the brick building and headed straight for the playground. On that second visit, they played and they played, staying so long that the heat of day softened into late afternoon, until the sky was a used-milk gray. John started to worry that maybe they'd stayed out too long, and his father would be looking for them.

"Been a long time," he said gathering June. "Let's find Dad."

John led his sister off the playground and back into the building. This time no one was there when they walked in. The office was empty. He looked around and for the first time noticed another room, off to the right, marked *Visitation*. Down a hall was a large dining room big enough for fifty people at least. Maybe more. John spun around looking for his father. Instead, he found a woman who told them, in a gentle but firm voice, that their father was gone and this—a strange place uncoupled from everything and everyone they'd ever known—was now their home.

John looked from the woman to his little sister, then to the front door and beyond. The truck was gone and, with it, their father. The room spun, and the world closed in. Heart pounding, tears welling, John realized with rising terror that his father had given them away. That's when the panic set in.

CHAPTER THREE

The Carrie Steele-Pitts Home was at 305 Roy Street in southwest Atlanta. Like the sixty-plus kids living there, it was tucked away on a quiet side street rarely visited by outsiders. Their ages and stories varied—some knew their parents; others didn't. They were all Black. For two kids who'd spent their entire lives in a tiny house, sleeping in bed every night with both of their parents, it was a massive and lonely place. For Clinton, it must surely have felt like the best of the bad options before him. For John and June, it was the end to everything.

They were immediately taken to separate dormitories, boys one way and girls the other. It would've been a traumatic experience even if they were together, but this break, one more in a series of breaks, was particularly hard on June. From the very beginning, the siblings began drifting apart. Still rattled and in shock, John was introduced to his new home. The cavernous dormitory where he and the other elementary school–aged boys would sleep atop steel bunks, the massive dining hall and common areas. He met his new house parents: three men with smiling faces and the impossible task of easing his transition. The hours passed in a fog until at last everyone was ushered off to bed.

It was a long night.

Morning, not just the next morning but every morning after, brought communal routine. The orphanage had a claustrophobic sort of togetherness. They did everything together. They woke as one, first making their beds and then heading to the bathroom to brush their teeth side by side at long sinks that held ten faucets each, and then crowded six at a time into the shower room. Each child had two sets of clothes, one to wear today as the other was washed, folded, and placed in identical piles at the foot of their identical beds. Any improperly made bunk whose blanket was rumpled or whose corners weren't tight enough had its sheets yanked off. They ate their meals together and, afterward, went to school together, sixty or more of them arriving at once in a noisy gaggle. Everyone at school knew them, collectively, as the orphans.

For all this physical proximity, for the inescapable closeness of their lives, the kids lived on emotional islands. At eight, John was scared and confused, craving more than anything a comforting touch or gently reassuring voice. He might as well have asked for his mother back. The kids were fed, clothed, and sheltered, never in need of necessities, but an orphanage isn't a family. There was little individual attention, few if any shared tender moments. There was no closeness, no hugs. No love. His house parents helped him, but he was one among many, and theirs would not be a parental relationship.

"I got thirty other kids to worry about," one of them said early on when they found John crying. "I can't spend time worrying about you being sad."

And so he kept it all inside. His first eight years had introduced him to hardship, but even then, in the chaos of a crumbling home amid unpaved streets, he'd been able to slip under the house and escape the world. Now he had nowhere to hide. He briefly considered running away, but the kids who'd tried were all quickly returned either by the police or by their parents—if they knew who and where their parents were and had made it that far.

He was given no choice. He was forced to adapt. It wasn't the worst life. There were other kids; he went to school for the first time; he even wore shoes. Hunger stopped being something he had to live with. None of which changed the fact that he'd been taken from his family and forced to stay here, where he was one among many. He felt tiny and tried to get even smaller by disappearing into himself. If he couldn't hide under the house, he'd hide in silence.

In the beginning his father would sometimes visit. These visits were sporadic and too brief when they happened, but it was something, a link to the life he'd known. Over time these stopped too. Not all at once but in drips, until one day the faucet was turned off.

John and June were called into an office, these two children slowly growing foreign to one another, where the news was delivered straight and without warning: "Your father died." That's how they were told. Not so much cold as matter of fact. They didn't attend the funeral. Through a bit of caprice or oversight they missed it. It would be years before they learned their father had tried and failed to get them back—a tragedy chalked up to Byzantine laws that barred parents from regaining custody once they surrendered it. Nor would they know how his health faded slowly, that he died alone and heartbroken. What John did know was that life was not his but something happening *to* him, and it made him feel small.

On that awful day, as the door to the room where they learned the news closed, John was told, "Come on back out when you're done." He stayed until all the emotion was gone.

THE CLOCKS THAT stopped the day his father died gradually began to tick again. John made friends and grew older. The orphanage, slowly, became home. On April 2, 1963, John's fourteenth birthday, two dollars arrived for him in the mail. He was beside himself. For the last seven years he'd never gone without, but then neither did he have anything to call his own. Every toy, meal, and moment had been shared with the other children, but this—these two crisp dollars bills—were his alone. It was almost too much. The other kids crowded around to look.

"Don't you touch it," he snapped. "This is mine."

John considered all the possibilities, but only briefly. "You spend this, you'll never have it again," he said to himself. So instead, he tucked it into an envelope that went everywhere with him. He slept with it under his pillow, hid it in his shoe when he showered, and carried it in his pocket when he went to school. He'd never had anything of his own before, and now that he did, he was determined not to lose it. He was far less determined to figure out who'd sent it. John's mind was everywhere and nowhere. He still preferred to be alone, and for that the radio was perfect.

Every soul singer in America—James Brown, Marvin Gaye, Aretha Franklin, name one—came through Atlanta, mostly playing places like the Royal Peacock, which was owned by a former circus performer. John never went there, never went anywhere, but the orphanage had a radio, which made it feel like they all came to him. His guy was Jackie Wilson, who had a string of hits—remember "Lonely Teardrops"?—an operatic voice, and an electric presence that had inspired both Elvis and James Brown. He was Mr. Excitement, all splits, spins, and backflips. He'd toss his jacket into the crowd and bring girls up to kiss him.

From the moment John first heard Wilson's music, it felt like magic. Alone by the radio, he practiced those dance moves—a frantic spin that tightened into a corkscrew, a dramatic drop to the floor, coat tossed over his shoulder. He couldn't do the splits, but that didn't matter. At the orphanage he had Jackie Wilson to himself, and really it was there, in solitude, that he drew comfort. You can't be ignored by the world if you ignore them first. Turns out, though, that you can't ignore the world—one day, the source of the money appeared, and his solitude was shattered.

Mary Kelly came from nowhere, just materialized unannounced. One moment John and June had nobody, no family, nothing at all, and the next they were being called into the visitation room to meet a woman they'd never seen who introduced herself as a distant cousin of their father's. Mary had learned of them from another cousin (also named Mary) who herself had learned of them from—it was complicated. John couldn't quite divine how he was related to Mary, either of them, but none of that mattered.

It was late spring, a season that in Georgia arrives on a sudden cloud of green pollen, a pink wave of azaleas. It's dramatic and beautiful but also short-lived. By the time Mary arrived, spring had already given way to summer, which set in like a wet blanket and smothered the breeze that might otherwise have blown in through the open window. The visitation room was hot. Mary outlined her own particulars—Pittsburgh housewife living with her husband, Robert, and four children, one of whom was grown and out of the house—then got to the point.

"I'm going to adopt you." There was silence. Before this moment neither John nor June had any reason to believe anyone might come for them. "You'll live with me. If you'd like to."

Once again life was happening to them. But at least it was happening.

CHAPTER FOUR

The trip from Atlanta to Pittsburgh took nearly two days by Trailways bus. Potholes and exhaust fumes, the soothing thrum of interstate monotony interrupted arbitrarily by stops in forgotten towns like Spartanburg and Gastonia, Wytheville, Beckley, and Weston. John slept when he could, which wasn't much, and spent the rest of the time watching the whole of Appalachia unfold before him. There, beyond his window, lay the first mountains he'd ever seen, an indication that his world was widening. Events inside the bus were far less dramatic.

Adoption was the miracle no one at the Carrie Steele-Pitts Home dared hope for, a surprise that for John required nothing but a simple "yes and where are we going?" And yet now that the day had arrived, all three of them, Mary included, were uncomfortable. What in their minds had played out as a joyous moment was, in reality, awkward. They didn't know each other. Conversation, stilted from the start, eventually waned and slowed to a trickle of necessity. Were they hungry or tired? Did they need to use the restroom?

Mary guided them onto one bus after another, each bringing them further from home. Staring out the window, John wondered what the kids back on Roy Street were up to. Once he caught sight of a wall-mounted clock and realized that all his friends were crowding into the dining hall for lunch. Even as he embarked on his new life, he couldn't let go of the one he'd left behind. He wondered if he'd ever see those kids again (he didn't) and if he'd miss them (he did). The orphanage had become home, what he knew and where he felt safe, and now he'd taken what felt increasingly like a blind leap of faith.

Probably Mary had apprehensions of her own. The decision to adopt John and June came against the advice of relatives who insisted the kids had been through too much and given too little, that they'd be unruly and wild, too big a burden for a middle-aged woman busy with a family of her own. She'd ignored that advice, but now, sitting beside two quiet children with big eyes and one-word answers, uncertain how they felt or how to coax anything from them, she must have wondered if she'd made the right decision.

The bus wound its way down the rolling hills, shuddered through a tunnel, and when it emerged, suddenly, Pittsburgh was everywhere. It was so much bigger than Atlanta, and louder. A river town dominated by steel mills and coke plants that scattered a dusting of red grit. The city teemed with railroads and streetcars, while its waterways were under siege from a flotilla of barges. It was a city of industry and of smoky air. There were rivers in all directions, each one breached at every conceivable point by yet another soaring bridge. For a child who'd come of age in an orphanage, it was incredibly intimidating. Like a moonscape.

ONCE IT GOT underway, family life was just as alien. Mary and Robert Kelley lived at 1719 Colwell Street, in a small brick row house with a white awning over the front steps. The kitchen was downstairs, below street level, with a little window that looked up at the sidewalk. They hung their clothes out back to dry and watched a black-and-white TV in the family room. All five of the children now living there slept in one of two bedrooms on the main floor. They went to church on Sunday—all day—and there were chores and rules. It was a lean operation, and they were accountable to each other.

Changes. Mary and Robert were no longer Mary and Robert but Mom and Dad. John's new father didn't say much. Late fifties, steelworker at the J&L Steel Company. Exhausted most of the time. He wasn't the kind of father to be out playing ball with the kids; usually he sat out on the back porch listening to a Pirates game on the radio. John's new brothers and sister were another challenge. William Hatch—the oldest, a veteran with psychiatric problems. Robert Kelley Jr.—younger than John, spoiled. Mary Pillows—recent high school grad on her way out. Clifford Pool—middle son, nicknamed Sonny, already gone.

The household itself was only the start. There was also an extended family: a whole army of aunts and uncles, cousins, grandparents, godparents. It was dizzying, all these people. They wanted to size him up, to shake, to hug and kiss, and make up for lost time.

"Come closer."

"Sit on my lap."

It was confusing and scary. Unnatural. He hadn't been hugged or kissed in longer than he could remember, didn't know how to be in a family, uncertain he wanted to learn, and now these strangers were trying to pull him close. School was just as bad. He started the eighth grade that fall. The teachers tried to stop him from entering, said an orphan from Georgia couldn't keep up (his accent didn't help—nobody understood him), and tried to get him sent away or at least back down a few grades. Under this shadow of suspicion, he showed up the first day in his best outfit—a blue sweater, red turtleneck, and grey pants. The kids made fun of the way he talked. When he showed up the next day in the same clothes (his best and *only*), they made fun of that too.

He'd been a neglected child and an orphan yet somehow never felt like he mattered less than he did now. In the Bottom everyone was poor; they all struggled. At the orphanage every child had been abandoned; they were all alone. Now he'd been taken in by a family where everyone had their place, his lowest of all. His father didn't really warm up to him. When he introduced him, he never called John his son or stepson but always "one of the kids Mary brought up from Georgia." His brother Robert did the same. And while John washed and folded his clothes each night, wore them again the next day, Robert Jr. had a closet filled to bursting.

The silence that defined his years in the orphanage gave way to resentment. He was angry. Began to ignore his siblings, break his parents' rules. Left the house without telling anyone where he was going or when he'd be back. He was grounded a lot, and his confinement was a punishment for everyone. His family didn't understand any of it. The psychology of grief and loss, the effects of untreated trauma, of yanking away everything a person loved, needed, and depended on—especially a child—weren't widely discussed or understood. It never occurred to anyone that John would be scarred by all the tumult, that adoption had arrived unexpectedly, amid a delicate phase of development, and that he'd be either unready or unwilling to move on.

Instead, most of John's family took his behavior as confirmation of their own suspicions. They'd tried to warn Mary, hadn't they? They knew this would happen. But she didn't listen, and now she was stuck with this angry boy. Most everyone simply threw up their hands. If John didn't want to be part of the family, then so be it. Let him stay on the side and sulk. Others thought maybe it'd be best to send him back to Georgia. Mary wasn't so stony; instead, she called in a counselor.

The first one failed to get through to him. The second, too. But they kept coming, one by one, each finding an angry teenager slumped at the table, annoyed at the intrusion and refusing to make eye contact. When they couldn't pierce his armor by gentle means, they switched to what could, very charitably, be called a tough love approach. In one meeting after another, they laid out the painful truth about his biological parents. The extent of Elzora's alcoholism. The details of how she'd died. They told John how Clinton had tried and failed to retrieve him from the orphanage, how he had died alone and lonely, just as he'd always feared he would. It was during these sessions that John learned his new family thought he'd be a burden and hadn't wanted him there, that they tried to convince Mary to leave him in the orphanage.

How anyone could have thought any of this would help is a mystery. Unsurprisingly, it only made him angrier and harder to handle because his anger was now joined by a sadness he could neither name nor express in any language but outbursts. One evening, after yet another of these painful sessions, John lay awake in bed staring at his lone outfit.

"Lord," John quietly prayed, "if you get me through this, I promise I will never rely on anybody for anything ever again."

CHAPTER FIVE

Magic. It had to be. It all changed so fast. A flash of light and his whole life turned around. Unless—maybe it was the prayer. Which would you believe, accident or providence, if everything, overnight, just got better?

John chose not to ask. In his second year with the Kelleys, ninth grade, he walked into Shep's Hardware Store on Fifth Avenue with a reference from his high school guidance counselor. He got a job stocking shelves—nothing that's supposed to change your life—but then came payday and for the first time he had money of his own to do as he wanted. And what the boy with one outfit wanted was clothes. All of them. From Shep's he'd hop the bus and hit Kaufmann's department store downtown, then go straight to Friedman's. The sales clerks knew him by name and gave him the run of the place. Alpaca sweaters and khaki pants, loafers in every color, gold jackets, blue pants—he said yes to everything. The more outrageous, the better. He spent every dime he made and never again wore the same clothes two days in a row. Basically never wore clothes twice, period. John strutted down Colwell Street as if he owned the place, his shoes gleaming in the sun.

Overnight his attitude improved—at home, school, everywhere. He got in less trouble; his grades went up; nobody laughed at him. Even made friends. They say the clothes make the man, and for the first time he could remember, John felt like somebody, like he mattered, and he thought this feeling would last forever. But reality was lurking just outside his door, a world that viewed him—regardless of how he dressed—a certain way, and he was old enough now that he began to see it clearly.

THE KELLEYS' HOUSE on Colwell Street sat in the Hill District, a neighborhood that had been known at various times as Farm Number Three, Prospect Hill, Arthursville, and Little Haiti. By the time John got there, everyone simply called it the Hill. Once owned by the grandson of the state's founder, William Penn, it was squeezed between the university and downtown. African Americans first arrived during the Revolution when the Continental Army began recruiting Black soldiers. After the war, those soldiers were joined by 150 freed men and women from Virginia, and together, in 1818, they founded the Bethel African Methodist Episcopal Church.

The refugees kept coming. Immigrants from Italy, Poland, Greece, and Germany. The Irish came, and so did European Jews. During the Great Migration, the Black population ballooned.

Harlem gets all the attention, but the Hill, a fraction of its size and geographically left of center, was the "Crossroads of the World." It was home to the *Pittsburgh Courier*, America's most influential Black newspaper, with a circulation of over four hundred thousand and star reporters like Evelyn "Big East" Cunningham—a six-foot-tall Black woman with red hair who hung out with Thurgood Marshall and covered lynchings and civil rights protests in every city, town, and backwater from Groveland to Birmingham. The Hill, a tiny hamlet, had two Negro League baseball teams, and one of them, the Crawfords, fielded one of history's great pitcher-catcher combos—Satchel Paige and Josh Gibson—and played in a lighted park before most of white baseball caught on to the idea.

August Wilson was from the Hill and would eventually set nine of his plays there, but it was jazz that made the neighborhood famous. Louis Armstrong, Dizzy Gillespie, Charlie Parker, Cab Calloway, and

Ella Fitzgerald all played there. Joe Louis hung out in the Hill. So did Lena Horne. The clubs became legend—Hurricane Lounge, the Ritz Club, the Flamingo Hotel, the Little Paris Club, the Blue Note, the Savoy Ballroom, the Pythian Temple. The most famous of them all was Gus Greenlee's Crawford Grill, which took up an entire city block. Music, dancing, and excess spread out over three floors, with a rotating stage on the second.

Although it was so many things, it was principally home. The Hill was a neighborhood of shop owners, mill workers, and the down and out. It had churches, grocery stores, five-and-dimes. But there was another side too. Slumlords owned much of it, and the city had allowed them to get away with code violations—egregious ones, almost criminal. Houses with flooded dirt cellars, buckling floors, rickety staircases, rusting fire escapes, and no heat. Houses with bad plumbing. Houses without plumbing. Garbage piling up around abandoned buildings. The Hill was the sort of place where you could get vegetables from a horse-drawn cart and Pirates games on the radio, but you could not, if you were Black and lived within its narrow borders, get a cab.

In the 1950s, Pittsburgh decided to shed its smoky steel town image and join the future. Urban renewal had a name here—Renaissance—and it would center around a $21 million plan to create a cultural acropolis on the edge of downtown. That there were people living on the site of this planned acropolis was seen as a minor detail. City councilman George Evans, who was white, said, "There would be no social loss if [the buildings] were all destroyed." The architect of Pittsburgh's Renaissance, Mayor David Lawrence, touted the "social desirability" of "complete clearance." *Urban renewal means Negro removal.*

The Hill's Black leadership wasn't opposed to change. Even major change. It wasn't just the decrepit buildings. Homes once built for a single family had been carved into apartments for two, three, or even four. The neighborhood was dangerously overcrowded. Tuberculosis and pneumonia rates were three times the city's average. Pittsburgh—a city that drained its municipal pools rather than desegregate them and was referred to as the "Mississippi of the North"—offered few apartments for Black renters and approved few loans for Black buyers. Homes were scarce.

Jobs more so. Echoing a common grievance, one man said US Steel would regularly "take a white man right out of the street and make you teach him and after you teach him, they give him your job or make him your foreman." Sensing an opportunity for advancement, Black leaders sought and received assurances that new housing would be built where old buildings were torn down and that all this work, the Renaissance, would bring jobs to the local community. With those promises in hand, they supported the project.

Work officially began on May 31, 1956, the same year John entered the orphanage. The first house to go, on Epiphany Street, dated back to the Civil War. The wrecking ball knocked it down and kept on swinging. The Old Bath House, a stop on the Underground Railroad, went down. So did all the jazz joints, including the Crawford Grill. A gothic church on Fernando Street—St. Peter's—came down, as did the Bethel AME Church. And all the houses went too. It happened so fast people hardly had time to leave. They stood on rooftops and watched their homes fall, often close enough to feel the ground shake.

Thousands of buildings were demolished. A triangle of land measuring one hundred acres was scraped completely bare. In its place went a civic center and office towers, condos. The Crosstown Boulevard was laid along the edge of the neighborhood. Meant to relieve traffic in the downtown triangle, it was designed by Robert Moses, whose New York City projects have often been criticized for hurting communities of color. Eight thousand people, 67 percent of them Black, lost their homes. But the fifteen thousand housing units promised under the deal never materialized. Nor did the work. The Hill got nothing. It was gutted, stripped of its culture and history. Its businesses were chased out, and its residents were piled into already overcrowded projects. City services, renovations, renewal, a great leap into the future—none of the Renaissance's promises ever materialized in what was left of the neighborhood. The Hill's pride and vitality, the music and celebrities, the shine were gone. In their place came poverty and hopelessness. Crime. Drug use. Reliance on public assistance.

John's family was among the lucky ones. Two parents, a stable income, their home left untouched. But he watched as all around him frustration turned into an impatient demand for change. People marched in the streets to protest discriminatory hiring practices at Duquesne Light, Bell Telephone, A&P, and the Pittsburgh Brewing Company. The NAACP was active locally, as was the United Negro Protest Committee and the Greater Pittsburgh Civic League. Martin Luther King Jr. spoke at the Pitt student union in 1966, and the next year Stokely Carmichael, chair of the Student Nonviolent Coordinating Committee, delivered a speech at the Hill's Ebenezer Baptist Church on the ideology of Black Power.

Approaching the end of high school, John shifted with the time. Gone were the loafers and alpaca sweaters. Inspired by Carmichael and Angela Davis, John wore a dashiki and started growing his hair out—the long march toward an afro. His parents didn't understand the look and were a little alarmed by its implications. He was only a few months from graduation, and they urged him to stay focused, assured him he would get everything he wanted if he worked hard enough. The world, they were quick to point out, had changed. It was April 1968.

CHAPTER SIX

The story broke just past seven p.m. on April 4. All three major networks interrupted their programming for a special bulletin. On CBS, Walter Cronkite anxiously shuffled a stack of papers before turning, stone faced, to the camera. "Good evening," Cronkite began in his deep rumble. "Dr. Martin Luther King, the apostle of nonviolence in the civil rights movement, has been shot to death in Memphis, Tennessee."

Eight hundred miles away, Pittsburgh slipped into a saddened state of shock. The city remained quiet through Thursday night and into Friday morning. It wouldn't stay that way when the shock wore off. Faculty at the Fifth Avenue High School urged John and his classmates, nearly all of them Black, to remain calm even as crowds gathered in the street to discuss what they should do. Sentiments were summed up pretty neatly by a guy who shouted, "They killed the most nonviolent member of the movement. Let's burn the place down."

A meat market on Centre Avenue was ransacked first, and from there it all unraveled. Florsheim's, the five-and-dime, Dickson Brothers Cleaners, the Mainway supermarket. People fought over shoes, meat, clothes, and stereo equipment. Practically everything moveable was either stolen or trampled underfoot. Signs like "Black Owned" or "Soul Brother Don't Burn Me Down" sometimes helped, but not always. Just the day before, in the hours after King was shot, police had maintained the fragile peace with an iron fist. They bashed a seventeen-year-old named Frank Cissell over the head with a nightstick just because he didn't get off the street fast enough. Now the tables had turned. Cops dispatched to the scene were taunted and pummeled with rocks. One officer grabbed his radio and screamed, "They're hitting everything!"

Then came the Molotov cocktails, an angry orange arc and the whoosh of air as buildings burst into flames. Rolling clouds of smoke. Grocery stores, shoe stores, a lumber yard—they all burned. Fire fighters were pelted with rocks. The area around Centre and Crawford, the heart of the Hill, was cordoned off by police. It was difficult to get out, impossible to get back in.

John was dizzy with anger and excitement when he reached Centre Avenue. Dusty shards of red clay from smashed bricks crunched under his shoes. The sky above was an eerie orange. For all his anger and frustration, violent outbursts were out of character for him. He lived in a house that revered authority. But he'd lived most of his life in one slum or another, had experienced segregation and racism, police brutality, poverty, and now emotion—pent-up for too long—came pouring out. It was violent and scary and a little mad—the entire Hill cutting off its own nose to spite someone else's face—but it was cathartic too. They had been ignored long enough. This time, surely, the world would have to listen. In the meantime, there would be violence and fires and, yes, looting. The roads would be paved over in spoiled food, broken windows, and a fine layer of ash.

On day three, four thousand National Guard troops arrived. Scores of them, like B-roll from Vietnam, lounging in the back of open transport trucks, chin straps dangling loose from their helmets. Looking out his windows, John saw soldiers manning .50-caliber machine guns in the back of olive-green jeeps. And so this was it. The moment of reckoning. Of being heard. Except it wasn't. The soldiers hadn't come for a fight. They came to make sure nothing happened to the business district or City Hall, to Squirrel Hill and all the other rich white neighborhoods. They were here to contain, to make sure whatever was happening in the Hill District stayed there, which meant that in the end this whole thing wouldn't matter, that Pittsburgh's Black residents and all their fury would remain unheard.

The violence, which climaxed on Palm Sunday and became known as the Holy Week Uprising, ended as abruptly as it started. The numbers were staggering. Five hundred fires, thirteen hundred arrests, well over half a million dollars in property damage. But the real toll was the sense of hopelessness left in its wake. Martin Luther King once called riots the "language of the unheard," and this sentiment seemed, in the days following the violence, a fitting epitaph for the people of the Hill. They'd burned the place down, and no one cared to hear why. What remained was an uneasy mix of sadness and anger, even shame, but also an energy one civil rights activist called "a fire in the belly." In a letter to the *Pittsburgh Post-Gazette*, local resident and Wesleyan College student Myrna Brown said the uprising was meant "to show that we are dissatisfied with our present condition . . . and that we are not going to settle for anything less than equal rights."

All the same, it shattered the sense of self John had gained from having a job and earning money of his own. Despite his hard work—six days a week—he was still a poor Black kid from the slums who didn't count for much. John felt as if fate's thumb was pressed down on his head. No matter how hard he tried, he couldn't rise.

He wasn't alone. The city of Pittsburgh wasn't alone. Since 1965, violence had flared up in one city after another as the cancer of hopelessness metastasized. If the questions were *why* and *how do we prevent the next one*, white America seemed to have no answers, though the answers, in many ways, weren't all that complicated if anyone cared to listen. So President Lyndon Johnson created an eleven-member commission to find some. Known as the Kerner Commission, it included senators and representatives, civic leaders, one chief of police, and the governor of Illinois, Otto Kerner. What they reported back—that recent violence in Black communities was rooted in racism, police brutality, and poor prospects for advancement—probably shouldn't have taken so long to find.

"What white Americans have never fully understood," the report declared, "but what the Negro can never forget, is that white society is deeply implicated in the ghetto. White institutions created it, white institutions maintain it, and white society condones it."

Nevertheless, John's parents didn't understand why he seemed so angry.

At dinners, he'd sit across from them, two generations frustrated and at odds over how best to proceed. They didn't understand the direction he seemed to be going, and John didn't understand why they weren't angry. So dinnertime was tense, the whole time his parents *tsking* over his hair and clothes, his attitude.

"Don't be doing all that stuff. I'm serious," his mother would say. "You gotta act right."

John would laugh, and that'd bring his father in. "It's not a joke. You don't act right, that white man's not gonna want you."

The first time John heard this, he looked up, surprised. His father stared him right in the eye.

"It's a white man's world, John. You gotta be the kinda Black guy the white man wants."

Silence. How else could he respond? As he saw it, his parents grew up in a world that forced them into submission, even now they couldn't muster the rebellious urge to stand up. They were trying to help. He knew that. And he felt sorry for all they'd been through, but this was a different time. His was a different generation, one that had seen the Civil Rights Act and the Voting Rights Act. The Fair Housing Act. They'd seen Freedom Riders, bus boycotts and garbage strikes and sit-ins. They grew up watching people face down police dogs, fire hoses, Bull Connor, and George Wallace: "Segregation now, segregation tomorrow, and segregation forever." Now they were being told to be patient, that change takes time, but they were through waiting. A rift had already opened in the civil rights movement. Disillusioned with the nonviolence preached by King, younger members like Carmichael—"My generation's out of breath. We ain't running no more."—had broken away from the older leadership. The same thing was happening across America. Even before the assassination, younger and more militant protestors in Pittsburgh had planned a "Burn Day" for May 1968. King's murder in Memphis sped up the timeline.

These disagreements, whether between national figures on a big stage or on Colwell Street between John and his parents, were endemic. The generational divide was wide and getting wider, and for people like John, change wasn't something to wait for but to go and make happen. And his generation—not content to be the kind of Black men somebody else expected—was going to make it happen.

He couldn't tell you how. Couldn't even tell you what change would look like. He knew only that it wouldn't just come to him, that he'd have to go out and grab it. After high school the search carried him away from Shep's and into the steel mills, and when he left there, it led him to the orderly training program at Montefiore Hospital. And that's where he was in the winter of 1971, twenty-two with a wife and son, looking for a way to make his mark on the world, when into his life walked two Black men in white jackets emblazoned with the word *paramedic*.

And just like that his moment had come.

CHAPTER SEVEN

John sat in a tiny office at Presbyterian-University Hospital—Presby—surrounded by silence. He shifted in his chair, then spoke.

"It's kind of like an obsession. You know?"

Across from him sat a man who said very little other than that his name was Will Holland. Just a few moments before, John had barged in and said he wanted to interview for a job with Freedom House, those words he'd seen on the paramedics' white coats. Holland grudgingly granted him one, and now John was blowing it.

Since the night he first saw them, John had been trying to figure out what a paramedic did (he still didn't know) and what Freedom House was (he had no clue), but at least he'd figured out where to find them. Another orderly told him they were headquartered at Presby, down by the ER, so John started going over there every night during his break. He didn't say anything—the medics themselves were too intimidating. He just stood on the edge of the shadows. Watched as they hung around outside, talking and smoking, driving off in their ambulances. He listened to the laughter and the cussing, the shit talk between people who've been through hell together and now have no boundaries.

To John, they didn't look like friends or coworkers but something else, closer to brothers-in-arms than brothers in fact. John wanted that badly. But he was intimidated. And in awe. So he didn't say anything. He just stood there, day after day. Watching. It was the ambulance that finally got him going. A two-tone Chevy G20 van, the kind of thing the ice cream man might drive. The top was painted white and bristled with lights, sirens, and a long whip antenna. The sides were orange with a large blue star of life plastered on its sliding door. The words *Freedom House* jumped out in large block letters. One night while he was there, the hospital doors swung open, and two medics rushed out. The ambulance tore out of the parking lot in a frenzy of red lights that bounced off the walls and reflected off John's glasses. It was loud and exciting, and it pushed John to make his move. As the ambulance disappeared down the road, he crossed the street and headed into the building. He realized very quickly he didn't know where he was going or who he was looking for, but that no longer mattered.

He opened doors and asked questions and poked around and eventually found himself, unbelievably, sitting in an office with a Freedom House supervisor. Will Holland, another Hill kid, wasn't much older than John, but he'd been at Freedom House since the beginning and had worked his way up. He stared at John now, waiting to hear something that would convince him that this guy who wandered in dressed like an orderly deserved a job. John started talking about obsessions.

"Since the first time I saw you guys, I knew this was what I was going to be. What I had to be."

Holland nodded.

"So I'd like an application," John said. Holland pulled a sheet from his desk drawer and handed it over. "I've been an orderly for a few years at Montefiore so I think I have the . . ."

John's voice trailed off. He hadn't been handed an application but a sketch of the human body, with an enlarged cutaway of the heart and lungs.

"What's this?"

Holland nodded at the paper. "You're able to identify the various parts of the heart and lungs, right?"

"Well, no. Not at all."

"I see." Holland took the paper back. "Then you're not qualified to work here."

John's heart sank. This was his shot, and he'd blown it. As he stood to leave, Holland called after him.

"Go get some training," he said. "You can't just come in off the street. You gotta be qualified to do this job."

John closed the door, walked out. Where was he going to get training? After all this, he still didn't even know—what the hell was a paramedic?

BOOK TWO

CHAPTER EIGHT

Hard facts first: paramedics give drugs; they diagnose (not really, but we're splitting hairs) and treat cardiac irregularities; they slip tubes into the lungs and breathe for anyone not breathing; they shock hearts that aren't beating. All this they do outside of the hospital, generally on an ambulance. They're often partnered with EMTs, who are skilled providers but have less training and cannot perform the advanced life support techniques that medics do.

Beyond their duties, paramedics represent an ideal. An assurance from society, backed by money, that human lives are sacred and will be saved anywhere and everywhere they're in danger. Society has often shrugged its burden and reneged on the deal. America pretended the burden didn't exist until 1965. But it's always been there.

Primitive versions of what you'd call a paramedic have been popping up in one country or another for much of history, always fizzling out and disappearing—sometimes for hundreds of years—only to remerge someplace else looking brand new. It's the falling cat that somehow lands on its feet.

Jesus made the earliest recorded reference to practicing medicine in the street. Gospel of Luke: A lawyer asks how to receive eternal life, and Jesus tells the story of the Good Samaritan. A man traveling from Jerusalem to Jericho gets attacked by bandits. Beaten, stripped, and left for dead. Several people, including a priest, see him lying naked but pass him by. Finally, the Samaritan comes along. He treats and bandages the man's injuries and then transports him on the back of a donkey to an inn so he can recover.

From there the story gets fuzzy, and whether the man lived or died, if the oil and wine helped or compounded his problem—who knows. We do know the promise of eternal life wasn't enough to convince people to start delivering medical aid at the scene of an emergency. That would take another twelve hundred years. Thirteenth-century Florence: A man named Pietro di Luca Borsi put a swear jar in the cellar where his friends gathered to drink. They were so numerous and so profane that the jar quickly overflowed. And kept on flowing. Before long, they had enough loose change to do with it something of significance. They settled on the unlikely decision to create a civilian ambulance service and called themselves the Brothers of Mercy. The Brothers covered themselves head-to-toe in heavy robes and carried the sick and injured to the hospital by hand on crimson litters. They were summoned by the tolling of a bell—one for common illness or injury and two for anything more serious. If the bell tolled three times, they'd essentially be carrying a hearse instead of a stretcher.

Eventually the Brothers faded away. Need for them remained, but the field never formalized. Others came and went. Taxis during the plague, horses during war. Despite *not dying* being the chief preoccupation of humankind, nobody put serious thought into creating a lasting service to deal with it. Until Napoleon.

Dominique Jean Larrey was born into obscurity in 1766, the son of a shoemaker from the French Pyrenees. At thirteen, Larrey was orphaned and sent to live with his uncle, overnight going from cobbler's kid to ward of the chief surgeon for the town of Toulouse. Guided by his uncle into a surgical apprenticeship, he showed a tremendous aptitude that eventually landed him a post in Napoleon's army. Larrey—who in civilian life would later perform mastectomies without anesthesia, a procedure patient Frances Burney described as terrifying "beyond all description"—was horrified by what he encountered on the battlefield.

The Napoleonic wars were long and brutal. Bullets, bayonets, grapeshot. Men dropping in columns, left to suffer and die where they fell. And no one did anything about it. Surgeons never got near the fight. No one was there to treat casualties or even decide who should get treatment and in what order. So Larrey devised a solution, and in 1797 he brought it to Napoleon: surgeons should be given the same nimble horse-drawn carriages that carried the army's "flying artillery" to use as ambulances. This way, rather than lying in misery and waiting to bleed out or die of infection, casualties could rapidly be transported to the hospital. He also proposed establishing a system to categorize the wounded by severity and transport those in need first. Napoleon liked the idea of saving rather than burying soldiers and said yes. In a single, brilliant stroke Larrey had invented not just the first dedicated ambulance corps but also the modern system of triage.

And for the next thirty-five years, the civilian world ignored it. Then came cholera.

Though it had existed in isolated pockets for centuries, cholera first made the leap to global pandemic in 1817. The outbreak started in the humid marshlands of India's Ganges Delta, sparked by contaminated rice. From there it followed European trade routes, spreading unchecked throughout the Indian subcontinent and across Asia. It's a nasty disease: the first symptoms—diarrhea and vomiting—come on suddenly and are joined shortly by severe abdominal cramps. The skin becomes shrunken with a distinctive bluish tint. Excessive fluid loss and septic shock lead to complete circulatory collapse and death. The whole thing takes only twenty-four hours. In its inaugural run, the disease raged through Thailand, Indonesia, the Philippines, China, and the Persian Gulf. Then it hit Turkey, Syria, and Russia before finally dying out in the harsh winter of 1823. It returned six years later, this time to stalk Europe.

When it reached the UK in 1831, cholera still had no identifiable cause or cure. People were terrified. It killed quickly and indiscriminately. Widespread fear of infection, along with anger over the government's inability to stop it, led residents to distrust Parliament and embrace conspiracy theories. Edicts from public health officials were seen as threats and ignored, while rumors that doctors admitted patients into the hospital just so they could kill and dissect them (something called Burking) spread almost as quickly as the disease itself. In some cities, the public rioted.

London's death toll—sixty-five hundred in 1832 alone—ratcheted up pressure on the medical community to do something. Its answer, so simple and effective it seemed obvious in retrospect, was to separate the infected from the healthy. At the first sign of symptoms, carriages set aside specifically for the purpose were dispatched directly to a patient's home, where they were loaded up and carted off to the hospital. Treatment remained guesswork, survival a crapshoot, but at least they weren't lying in a crowded apartment infecting everyone around them. Though cholera would resurface, the world's first hospital-based ambulance service had shown Europe how to contain it.

America was another story. On January 9, 1861, a college student named G. E. Haynsworth fired a cannon at the *Star of the West*, a Union supply ship steaming through Charleston Harbor. It was the opening shot of the Civil War. It was also the birth of the American ambulance. A few years prior, Britain had sparked a global controversy during the Crimean War by failing to field a military ambulance service. Casualties were massive. It was covered in American papers, and US generals were there to witness it. But they failed to learn the lessons, and in 1861, armies of the North and South both staffed their puny ambulance corps with men "of the lowest character."

In 1862, Henry Ingersoll Bowditch volunteered to serve as a surgeon with the Union army and was shocked by what he found. Wounded men left on the battlefield for days. Ambulance crews stopping to pillage farmhouses. Drivers falling drunk from the wagons.

"The scarcity of ambulances," he wrote to the surgeon general, "the want of organization, the drunkenness and incompetency of the drivers, the total absence of ambulance attendants are now working their results." Bowditch's own son, a second lieutenant shot through the jaw, died lying in the field and waiting for help.

Heartbroken and enraged, the fiery abolitionist had a new crusade. Bowditch took his ambulance fight to anyone who would listen, and many who wouldn't, eventually penning a passionate missive titled, in part, "A Brief Plea for an Ambulance System." Widely disseminated, "A Brief Plea" struck a chord in Washington and helped spur a reluctant Congress to create the country's first organized ambulance system. Since none existed—and the war was still raging—it would have to be built. Fast. Cincinnati, a town whose pork-based economy shriveled during the war, leading its factories to sit idle, stepped into the breach and became the nation's largest producer of ambulances.

After the war, with unused ambulances sitting around, Cincinnati became the home of America's first civilian ambulance service. These were primitive things, horse-drawn and incredibly uncomfortable. No equipment, no doctors or trained medical personnel. Their first driver, a man named James Jackson, was paid $360 a year to sling patients around the city. For a moment, Cincinnati was on the cutting edge. Then New York took over.

NINETEENTH-CENTURY NEW YORK was crowded and chaotic, prone to violence, industrial accidents, and the odd bout of cholera. But Edward Barry Dalton, a former regimental surgeon newly hired as New York's sanitary superintendent, developed a cure: a brand-new, hospital-based ambulance system that would one-up London, Cincinnati, and anything else the world had ever seen. It took some doing, but he convinced the city, and on June 4, 1869, Dalton's ambulances hit the streets.

The system was innovative but complex. It started with the police. Alerted to an emergency, a beat cop would fire off a telegraph to the eighteenth precinct—neighbor to New York's infamous Bellevue Hospital—with the nature and location of the emergency. A runner from the precinct would grab the dispatch and sprint to Bellevue's front gate to request an ambulance. Deep inside the bowels of the hospital, a horse would be hitched, the two-man crew readied, and out into the streets the whole team would race.

In the beginning, Bellevue had just two drivers, Daniel McGuire and James Stone, who were each paid $30 per month to be on standby all day every day. Together, driver and horse were the brains and brawn behind this state-of-the-art machine. It was seven feet of wood painted a gleaming black with crisp canvas sides, the whole thing lit by oil lamps that swung from the corners. There was a foot-powered gong mounted up front to scatter crowds, while the floor in the back—doubling as a stretcher—was specifically designed to slide out.

This alone set the curve, but Dalton took it a step further. Each ambulance would also carry an array of medical equipment. Tourniquets, splints, blankets, straps for immobilizing fractures, bandages, sponges, a two-ounce bottle of persulfate of iron (for bleeding) and a quart flask of brandy (for everything else). Over time, a straitjacket was added to the kit. The final stroke of genius, perched jauntily on the back, facing sideways and bracing himself against the opposite side with his feet, was perhaps Bellevue's greatest innovation: a doctor.

By the end of the year, the service had run 558 calls—everything from suicides and explosions to a man who'd been tossed from a third-story window by his wife. New Yorkers slowly grew accustomed to the sight of black Bellevue ambulances racing by in a clatter of gongs and thundering hooves, leaving in their wake startled onlookers and the lingering scent of lamp oil and wood varnish. In its first few months, Bellevue crews lost only four patients during the cross-city ride to the hospital. Calls grew more frequent as people who previously had no access to health care suddenly had doctors rushed right to their side free of charge.

There were issues along the way, the whole thing grew in fits and starts, but from here emergency medicine began to move very quickly. It remained, however, the domain of men.

In 1849, Elizabeth Blackwell had become America's first female physician, yet fifty years later it was only the rare woman who joined her. Those who did were generally restricted to treating women and children, but in 1901 a doctor named Emily Dunning bucked the trend by convincing New York officials to let her test for the position of ambulance surgeon. The job was considered prestigious by then, and she was matched against some of the country's best young doctors—all of whom she outperformed by placing first on the exam. Still she was refused a job. But Dunning didn't give up. She fought the hospital board, took her case to the mayor, and finally, in July 1903, a full two years after acing the exam, became the first female ambulance surgeon.

Her first call was for a peanut vendor whose right leg got crushed beneath the wheel of a brewery truck. Reporters followed Dunning to the scene, where she stabilized and splinted the vendor's leg—badly broken, the bone jutting out from the skin—and got him loaded and off to the hospital so quickly that a cop watching the whole thing turned to a reporter and said, "She'll do."

Across the country, Bellevue's system was borrowed from and altered liberally. Not always for the better. Cleveland's ambulances were based out of funeral homes, and morticians quite literally caught people going and coming. Rochester, Seattle, and Los Angeles turned to the police. In San Francisco, then still a wild and exotic dot on the Barbary Coast, patients were taken to drugstores, the most famous of which—the Port of Broken Heads—treated a half dozen or more patients every night of the week.

Then the nascent field received a push by necessity. The year 1914 marked the start of World War I, one of history's great meat grinders, which advanced ambulance technology further in just a few years than all the previous centuries combined. Mounted cavalry charges and open-field advances were met with mustard gas, artillery, planes, and machine guns. In just one day at the Somme, fifty-seven thousand British troops were killed or wounded. That battle was no anomaly. The question of what to do with all these causalities arose, and in the scramble to save and reuse the Allied wounded, America—officially neutral until 1917—lent a much-needed hand.

The Ford Motor Company donated Model Ts to be repurposed as ambulances, as did philanthropists like the Vanderbilts, and scores of young Americans—twenty-five hundred by the end of the war—volunteered to drive them. They bounced along bombed-out and darkened roads, picking up the wounded within reach of the front lines. It was dangerous work. Ernest Hemingway, who drove a Red Cross ambulance in Italy, was injured by shrapnel and spent months convalescing in an Allied hospital, an experience he turned into *A Farewell to Arms*.

When the US joined the fight in 1917, the army's medical department took this early ambulance work a step further, assigning a unique pair of enlisted men to each company stationed on the Western Front. Trained in first aid, these troops treated the injured right in the trenches, a shift in thinking that became the first-known use of medics anywhere in the world. While this on-the-scene treatment greatly improved the chances of survival, it marked just the first step in a newly designed tiered system of care. After medics stabilized the wounded, they were carried to a company aid station for further treatment—including tetanus shots—before being transferred to a battalion aid station. There they were evaluated, treated, and loaded into ambulances for transport to definitive care at a field hospital.

By 1918 ambulance medicine had made a quantum leap. The advent of two-way radio communication sped the delivery of care, which by the war's final days even arrived by plane. Traction splints—medieval-looking devices that pulled apart and stabilized the jagged ends of a broken femur—proved remarkably effective at saving lives.

As did the medics themselves. Selected directly from the ranks of soldiers, medics spent ten weeks learning to splint fractures and dress wounds. They learned to recognize and treat trench foot and how, under supervision, to give morphine. This brief and hyperfocused education meant medics could be trained in much higher numbers than doctors and placed right in the middle of the action.

After the war, all this knowledge, equipment, and personnel returned home. Ambulance service in the US seemed poised to flourish as never before.

And it did. For a minute. Municipalities that could afford them established paid ambulance services, and volunteers stepped in for many that couldn't. Even as the ambulance surgeon was slowly replaced by the cheaper and more plentiful ambulance technician, the field remained attached to local hospitals and maintained a reasonable standard of care. But America was growing and changing, and the ensuing decades were marked by upheaval that once again stunted the growth of its emergency medical services.

Hospitals were the first link in the chain to break. Between 1934 and 1949, hospital admissions rose by a total of ten million patients, placing the health system under a tremendous strain that only got worse with the outbreak of World War II. As the war effort ramped up, hospitals were hit hard by rationing. They were short on doctors, supplies, and funding. Those institutions that still maintained an ambulance service quickly dumped it.

Overnight, the ambulance transformed from a medical service into a municipal one, as police and fire departments grudgingly picked up the slack. It never truly fit in either place and was treated like a Frankenstein limb rather than a full-fledged arm of public safety. The ambulance was all but ignored by police departments, which were focused on the nation's rising crime rate, while among firefighters ambulance duty was regarded as a form of punishment. The song was much the same across the swathes of America still relying on funeral homes for emergency care. Running a medical call required use of a hearse and two morticians but brought in only a fraction of what a funeral did. For budget-conscious mortuaries, transporting the living became little more than an advertisement for the inevitable—and much more lucrative—last ride of the dead.

Regardless of who was providing it, emergency medical services suffered from an unwillingness to invest either the time or the money required to keep technicians sufficiently trained and equipped. And in the absence of state- or federally mandated standards, *sufficient* became a term loosely interpreted at the local level to mean the absolute bare minimum. By the 1950s—nearly a century after Bellevue had assigned surgeons to the job—the American ambulance was staffed by attendants with all the expertise of a lifeguard at the public pool.

That this decline occurred simultaneous to the military medic's rise in prowess and stature threw the problem into stark relief. In World War II, shouts of "Corpsman!" echoed across the European and Pacific theatres, while soldiers and surgeons alike returned from Korea with the knowledge that their lives and careers had been saved by corpsmen. The medical community was well aware of the corpsman's potential, but efforts to create a civilian analog were met with indifference. The field hadn't just stalled; it'd gone backward. And it showed. After a 1956 train derailment in Los Angeles, competing ambulance companies were so busy fighting one another over who would transport the injured that the victims were transported instead in private vehicles. This might've been scandalous if anyone really cared. A survey conducted a few years later revealed that only 22 percent of US cities regulated ambulances, and only 8 percent required advanced first aid training to work on them. On any given day, the patient in an ambulance may have been better qualified to handle their own emergency than the person paid to save them. By the 1960s, preventable deaths had become a public health crisis.

In 1965, forty-nine thousand Americans died in car accidents, more than were killed in the entirety of the Korean War. Many of these deaths were considered preventable with the right combination of automotive safety standards and emergency medical response, and this fact, along with the sheer number of fatalities, prompted passage of the Highway Safety Act in September 1966. As that bill was making its way through Congress, the National Research Council published a thin pamphlet called "Accidental Death and Disability: The Neglected Disease of Modern Society." Known simply today as the White Paper, it made a lot of accusations and suggestions, though the thrust of it could be boiled down to a simple truth: ambulance technicians were too few to be there when needed, and too unskilled to be of much use when they arrived.

Just how few and unskilled? According to the White Paper, things had gotten so bad that an American shot in Vietnam was more likely to survive than if he'd been shot right here in the States. The reason for this was simple: the soldier had a corpsman crouching over him. The civilian had no help at all. Those are the kind of incendiary facts that should've turned 1966 into a watershed moment for street medicine. And it almost did. Instead, Washington, which had already tasked the Department of Transportation with improving highway safety standards, now added to this burden the job of elevating the medicine practiced on ambulances to a level somewhere above lethal.

The DOT may seem a strange band of bureaucrats to trust with medical advances, but they gamely set to work, issuing a decree that highway funds would only go to states that created an effective ambulance system (the same tactic Congress leveraged again twenty years later to get the drinking age changed). This was a good start. But they never made good on the threat. Nor did they define what *effective* meant. Or suggest minimum standards for training and equipping this medical force or even who would pay for it. Instead, everything was left to local officials, the very people whose indifference created the current crisis and who time and again had let the blueprint for street medicine slip through their fingers. Nevertheless, the White Paper set some very slow moving wheels in motion, and eventually, years down the road, action did follow.

But for now, no clear path had been set, and no true rewards or punishment existed for those who followed or strayed from it. So things carried on as they always had. Fixing this would require untangling a century of antiquated and ineffective methods and replacing them with something politicians instinctively identified (and avoided) as expensive. And even if you had the money, did you have the ability, the stamina, the right mix of genius and hubris and hard-headedness to actually pull it off? Mostly the answer was no. But one person did, and history had put him on a collision course with Freedom House.

CHAPTER NINE

On the night of November 4, 1966, five years before John's disastrous interview, staff arriving at the Presby ER for the nightshift shook off the cold and fell into the addled rhythm of a busy city hospital waiting for the crush and chaos of Friday night to begin. There, among the doctors and nurses, the assortment of patients in varying degrees of need, one presence stood out. Dressed in a white lab coat and threadbare pants, hovering over charts at the nurses' station, was a fast-walking anesthesiologist named Peter Safar.

Safar was Austrian, with a nasally and slightly clipped Viennese accent that had not appreciably mellowed since he emigrated to the US back in 1949. He was slightly built, with a dark head of wavy hair framing a face that broke frequently and easily into a big smile. However fast Safar walked—and it was fast—he thought and, for that matter, drove even faster, his every movement the expression of an intense and probing intellect. His was a restless mind.

At just forty-two, Safar had already lived out a legendary career in medicine. While working at Baltimore City Hospital in the 1950s, he studied the existing methods of resuscitation and deemed them useless. So he created his own. Safar developed the technique we now call mouth-to-mouth and paired it with chest compressions, single-handedly revolutionizing how medicine treated—and saved—someone with no pulse but whose heart had stopped recently enough for their body to be salvageable. The medical community would call this type of patient "clinically dead." By 1966, his technique was being taught not only to medical professionals but also to lifeguards and teachers, parents, waiters, anyone. It was an unprecedented public health effort that would save millions of lives. Known forever-after as the Father of CPR, Safar could've retired on the spot and been considered a wild success.

But he didn't. Instead he accepted an offer to join the University of Pittsburgh health system and establish an anesthesiology department. Medicine was his calling. In between creating and staffing this new department, he also pulled shifts in the ICU and the ER, recruited and mentored medical fellows, and also in his spare time attended to the varied obligations of a father and husband—which included (naturally) dominating the city's annual waltzing competition with his wife, Eva. His was a full schedule, but Safar was restless, and his thousand-mile-per-hour pace left room for the occasional side project. In the fall of 1966, that project was to sketch out the parameters of a state-of-the-art emergency medical service.

That this had eluded the collective minds of modern medicine didn't in any way discourage Safar. His budding obsession with prehospital medicine was personal, tied to a haunting tragedy, and its success had become an imperative. Safar's ideas extended well beyond the simple training and equipping of ambulance technicians and went so far as to prescribe the specific capabilities and precise dimensions of the ideal ambulance. And he was happy to share them with anyone who would listen. The problem was nobody would listen. Yet.

Around seven thirty on the night of November 4, as Safar worked the Presby ICU, Pittsburgh Democrats were gathering just a few blocks away at an event and concert hall known as the Syria Mosque. Built in the city's Oakland neighborhood for the Masonic society known as the Shriners in 1916, the enormous brick structure was four stories of exotic revival architecture, complete with a pair of eleven-foot-long bronze sphynxes guarding the front entrance. The ornate auditorium was so big that the twenty-five hundred people in attendance on this cold Friday in November barely filled half of it. The crowd was raucous.

On Tuesday, Pennsylvania would elect its next governor, and the rally was intended to kick off a weekend of furious campaigning and help deliver a victory for the Democratic candidate, Milton Shapp. At eight pm, politicians and dignitaries from around the state filed into their front-row seats, and the rally got underway. Despite rumblings of a rift within the party, the mood was high that night, as the speakers rose in turn to address the crowd. Thirty minutes into the program, David Lawrence—a former governor and four-term mayor of Pittsburgh, the aging lion of the state's Democratic Party—stood for his turn to speak.

At seventy-seven, Lawrence, architect of the Renaissance, was still robust, the sort of politician forever photographed throwing out a first pitch. His image—characterized by round, wire-rimmed glasses and graying hair neatly combed back—was everywhere. Lawrence had helped wrench western Pennsylvania from Republican hands, creating in the process a powerful political machine that within the decade would put Democrats in control of the entire state. He was beloved. Especially here.

Standing below the stage, Lawrence grabbed the lectern with both hands and stared out at the assembled crowd. He was an experienced and seasoned speaker, and rather than preparing a full speech, he'd simply jotted down a few words on the back of an envelope. Words like *fear, suspicion, reaction. Progress, labor, human welfare, Medicare, civil rights*. These terms he felt delineated the difference between the two parties. He never got to say them. Almost as soon as he started speaking, his voice weakened and trailed off.

Though no one yet knew it, something was gravely wrong with David Lawrence. Without warning, he toppled backward into the stage, carrying the lectern with him as he went. Then he surged forward again—still holding the lectern—and stammered, "I'm fainting." Either that or he said, "I've never seen the Democratic Party more united," repeating the word *united* as he slumped over. Opinions differed. It seems unlikely he said much of anything. He teetered only briefly before collapsing to the ground, and from there he never spoke again.

Several men in the front row jumped up. State Secretary of Internal Affairs Genevieve Blatt knelt beside him to pray. Behind her, witnesses would remember an "almost visible shock" passing through the crowd. Someone in the audience rushed off to call an ambulance, while a man crouching over Lawrence loosened his collar and yelled for a doctor. Karen McGuire, a twenty-two-year-old nurse who had turned out for the rally, began pushing through the crowd. By the time she reached the governor, he wasn't breathing. McGuire tilted his head back, pinched off his nose, and delivered a rescue breath.

The audience was stunned into a terrible silence. A short while later—minutes in reality, but for McGuire weeks, months—a commotion rose from the back of the auditorium. Help had arrived. Or at least its only available approximation. Cops worked the ambulance in Pittsburgh. The distress call placed after Lawrence's collapse had gone out to the city police dispatcher, who raised a two-man police ambulance crew.

Most of the officers working on the department's medical wagons were long-serving veterans who hadn't taken a first aid course in years. Any knowledge they hadn't forgotten had likely slouched into malpractice through decades of poor habits. And if they knew little, they were equipped with even less. Pittsburgh's police ambulances, clunky old trucks known colloquially as Black Betties, carried little more than a stretcher. Cops didn't stabilize or even treat patients, just rushed them to the nearest hospital. Their doctrine of haste began the moment they reached Lawrence.

McGuire was still doing mouth-to-mouth when the cops tossed a canvas cot down by her side. She tried to put Lawrence on oxygen, but the cops' cannister was either empty or broken. It almost didn't matter because from here all semblance of order fell apart. McGuire was shoved aside. The cops snatched Lawrence and tossed him onto their stretcher. Then they were up and moving back through the crowd. McGuire tried her best to keep up, but the cops were frantic to get outside. Lawrence was bull-rushed toward the door, flopping around on the stretcher, his skin rapidly turning an ominous shade of cadaver white.

McGuire made an attempt at mouth-to-mouth while stumbling along, but the cops' speed wouldn't allow it. The crowd followed the stretcher as it bumped through the doors and out into the icy chill of the night. The cops stopped to yank open the doors of their wagon, giving McGuire just enough time to check on Lawrence and find he no longer had a pulse. This was neither of interest nor concern to the cops. They shoved the stretcher in and started to close the doors. For all intents and purposes Lawrence—one of Pittsburgh's most famous politicians—was dead, and neither of the two city employees sent to rescue him even considered riding in the back to help. McGuire forced her way inside before the doors slammed shut.

Back inside the Syria Mosque, the crowd was shaken and a little queasy. They observed a moment of silence. They knew something bad had just happened but not that the worst wasn't over. At that very moment, the cops were driving so recklessly to the hospital that McGuire was being thrown around the ambulance, unable to provide care. In a situation where every second counts, entire minutes ticked away.

Dr. Campbell Moses, Lawrence's personal physician, would later point to this prolonged period in which Lawrence received little to no treatment as the crucial factor in the former governor's death. Without oxygen, brain tissue rapidly begins to die. This is what happened to Lawrence, and the resulting brain damage, Moses concluded, was what killed him. "If we could have reached him three minutes earlier," he said, "it could've been a different story."

But the Democrats who looked to Lawrence as their de facto leader weren't outraged by what they'd just witnessed because they didn't realize that it was something on the level of a crime. That Lawrence's only chance for survival had been squandered by the sorry state of ambulance care in a city he'd devoted his life to serving. They didn't know any of this.

But Safar did. And as the ambulance screeched up to Presby, the Father of CPR was waiting at the entrance.

CHAPTER TEN

The elements that made Safar the ideal person for this moment originate an entire ocean and half a century away. He was born in Vienna on April 12, 1924, to two doctors, Vinca and Karl, who met in medical school while dissecting bodies. They were bohemians, avid alpinists, committed pacifists. Being an outlier was a genetic condition. Safar and his younger sister, Hanni, grew up with music and art. Their parents debated politics and discussed medicine; they took the kids hiking, skiing, ice skating, swimming in alpine lakes. Idyllic from a distance but far from perfect. World War I cost Austria its empire and left the country mired in an economic depression so deep even a two-doctor household could rarely afford meat. Worse times were on the way.

On March 11, 1938, Safar and his father went to the Vienna opera house to hear a performance of Tchaikovsky's *Eugene Onegin*, featuring celebrated Czech actress and soprano Jarmila Novotna. When it was over and the last note had drifted into the ramparts, they stepped outside to find the world had changed. The Ringstrasse, Vienna's historic boulevard, was thronged with crowds waving swastikas and chanting "communists . . . socialists . . . Jews—perish!" Safar was startled and confused. His father wasn't. While they were inside enjoying the opera, German troops had flooded across the border to begin the Nazi annexation of Austria. Within two days, Hitler's army occupied Vienna and remained there until the end of the war.

Life unraveled quickly. Now that they were in control of the country, the Nazis demanded all Austrians provide documentation of their ancestry. Vinca's showed that she was half-Jewish. The Nazis deemed her a Mischling, a slur that roughly meant "mixed thing." She was fired from her job. Karl lost his for refusing to join the Nazi Party or return its salute. Life was growing more dangerous—especially for young Peter.

At thirteen he was conscripted into the Jungvolk, a prelude to the Hitler Youth. He quit and was summoned to the local office of the Gestapo but ultimately, as the child of a Mischling, was excused. After high school, he was sent to a labor camp, where he dug ditches outside Munich. After several months he was released and promptly drafted into the army. Safar trained as a telegrapher and was slated for the Russian campaign, which by 1942 had become a death sentence. Here fate intervened and saved his life. While home on leave, Safar was caught in a heavy rainstorm that soaked his uniform. The wet wool irritated his skin so badly that he broke out—from waist to neck—in a raging case of eczema severe enough to get him hospitalized. His parents' friends went to work.

For the next few months, a series of friendly doctors surreptitiously kept him on the patient rolls even after his skin had cleared up. They did this at great personal risk, putting their own lives on the line each time Safar was juggled from one hospital to another, always just a step ahead of the SS inspectors. It was a difficult trick to maintain, and the entire thing nearly collapsed in the spring of 1943, when a surprise inspection threatened to out him. With no time to get away and fearing immediate deployment to the front—if not summary execution for desertion—Safar smeared his entire body with a caustic ointment that produced a reaction so violent it could've killed him.

But it worked. When the Nazis arrived, rather than an able-bodied young man available to fight and die in Stalingrad, they found only a sick patient. Safar was given a medical discharge at last. Freed from the threat of Nazi conscription, he restarted his studies. As John Moon would do a few decades later, Safar worked as an orderly in the city's General Hospital. They were hectic, contradictory days. One day Safar would be huddled at home dodging Allied bombs, and the next he'd be helping treat those who weren't so lucky.

In April 1945, Vienna's General Hospital became the center of a pitched battle between the advancing Russian army and SS troops holding the line. At one point, the SS tried to storm the hospital and use it as a fortress. Staff had already tipped over a bus to block the courtyard, but now soldiers were at the door. To keep them out, a senior physician named Leopold Schönbauer put on a general's uniform and ordered the soldiers to leave. Shockingly, it worked: they turned and walked away, leaving the hospital neutral but still in the middle of the fight. In the coming weeks, Safar and his coworkers would repeatedly—and under sniper fire—dash outside in their white coats to drag the wounded in for treatment.

Finally, on April 12, 1945, the curtain that had fallen over Austria was lifted. Russian troops marched into the capital city as liberators. One of those liberating soldiers happened to wander into the courtyard of Vienna's General Hospital, and there he came across Safar, exhausted and elated. The two young men, both irrevocably marked and changed by years of conflict, shook hands before going their separate ways. It was Safar's twenty-first birthday.

Within two months, he was back at Vienna Medical School. He graduated amid the rubble of a broken continent on March 19, 1948, and went to work on a ward for patients with severe burns and open wounds. Mostly that meant he kept people comfortable while they died.

One of the philosophies that would color his work began to emerge during this time. It would lead to great breakthroughs but also huge dustups. Safar was rebellious. Having survived the deadliest war in human history—some seventy million lives sucked into a vortex that arrived at his doorstep first—Safar adopted the philosophy that even one more death was too many. So he ignored any rule, norm, or formality that didn't save lives.

This showed itself quickly. Safar was a surgical intern under Dr. Schönbauer, the man who just a few years before had stared down SS troops trying to storm the hospital. Schönbauer was now the director of the hospital and Austria's first neurosurgeon. He was a giant, especially in Vienna, where his word was law. Perfect conditions for Safar to begin his rebellion.

As head of the hospital, Schönbauer led daily rounds and required all students and interns to follow behind him in a line snaking through massive patient wards that spanned a full city block. Safar couldn't stand it. The rounds took too long, and he learned too little. So he stopped going. Just skipped it. The first time Schönbauer arrived at a bed to find Safar already there instead of trailing behind and listening in on rounds, he was furious. Schönbauer stared at this young trainee with absolute rage but never said a word. And neither did Safar, who did the same thing the next day. And the next.

Vienna had become too small, and Safar wanted out. He needed to escape the Old World, leave behind the rules and rigidity of European medicine for someplace new and advanced and more promising. In September 1949, he was offered a surgical fellowship at Yale and accepted without hesitation. The boy from Vienna would become a citizen of the world.

Safar reached New Haven, Connecticut, without a dime in his pocket, wholly reliant on the $30 monthly stipend provided as part of his fellowship. Even if he managed to find a free place to stay, and he eventually did, $30 didn't even buy enough to eat. So he found a side job translating papers and then a second, more dangerous job mounting TV antennas atop New England's notoriously steep and slippery roofs. He now had enough money to buy food, but it was the unexpected arrival of a $75 check—mailed from a man in Miami who owed money to his father—which allowed him to buy a used car. Very used. So used it threatened to fall apart at any moment.

In class he was thrilled to find American professors not only allowed but encouraged disagreement. On campus, debate seemed half the point, and the medicine was more advanced as well. In Austria, anesthesia meant placing an ether-soaked rag over a patient's nose and smothering them out of consciousness. In the United States, patients were knocked out by IV medication and then intubated with rigid rubber tubes so a physician could deliver precisely the right amount of oxygen during surgery. It was all new and exciting, and it was around this time that he learned of the possibility of practicing anesthesiology as a specialty. It was a brand-new field and rapidly growing. He could already see that it had tremendous promise, and for the right doctor coming along at the right moment, it would provide freedom as well as the greatest chance to advance medicine and save lives. The field and the physician were tailor-made for each other.

Safar shifted his focus from surgery and never looked back. In the spring of 1950, he was twenty-six and on his way. But he was also single. He'd met several women in America but found them too puritanical for a young man who just a few months prior had been running loose in the euphoria of postwar Vienna. And anyway he remained fascinated by the memory of a beautiful and mysterious woman he'd met before leaving. In June, he braved a second north Atlantic crossing to go get her.

A RASCAL. THAT'S how Eva's cousin Milus Kalbac described Peter Safar. He was a rascal, mischievous, the kind of rambunctious boy who teased everyone, including his grandmother. Eva Kyzivat didn't know anyone like that and certainly wasn't supposed to date anyone like that. But she wanted to.

When the war started, Eva was only eleven. She spent her formative years fleeing to one or another of the city's air raid shelters, emerging after the all clear to see if her house had survived (it did, but the family's jewelry store was eventually destroyed). Her education was routinely interrupted, her childhood a blur. At seventeen she was naïve and inexperienced, the product of a decade lived in suspended animation. But it was 1947 now, and her cousin Milus—a medical student six years older—had invited her to a dance. This boy, the mischievous Peter, was going to be there, and Eva couldn't say no.

She hopped on a trolley, but Vienna was in the midst of rebuilding, and the lines took her only a few blocks. She got off and walked the rest of the way. Since the end of the war, she'd started skiing, hiking, listening to music, and dancing, but life was opening very slowly, too slowly for the older kids. Milus didn't want Eva to miss out. When they arrived at the party, Eva was the youngest and the only one not in medical school. She was nervous until Milus introduced her to Peter. She knew right away she was in trouble.

Safar too. The music played, but the world fell away, leaving nothing but this young woman and the shy smile that wrinkled her nose, and he knew as he stood there he was in love. Maybe that was cliché, but who cared? The war was over, and somehow they'd made it. They were alive in this moment, and everyone was dancing. They danced all night.

They started dating right away. They went to concerts; they rode bikes and took walks in the woods. Eva realized that however mischievous Safar was, he had a serious side too. Unlike the other boys she'd dated, he was idealistic and philosophical, a busy medical student who'd put deep thought into any number of topics. He was also driven in a way she'd never seen. He never said it, and she didn't ask, but she sensed his obsession with making something of himself was a sort of penance for having survived the war. She sensed, too, that he would accomplish the grand plans he'd made for himself, that he'd get out of Vienna and see the world, maybe even save the world, and she wanted to be there for it.

News of his fellowship and impending move to the United States, then, came as no surprise. When he left, she kissed him goodbye and continued with her life. She had to finish school, and besides, there were other boys in Austria. She dated several but found it harder and harder to deny that Peter was the love of her life. They spoke only in letters until June 17, 1950, when Safar stepped off a train in Vienna. Eva was there to meet him. They drove to an overlook called Leopoldsberg, and he asked if she would join him in America.

With her shy smile, the wrinkled nose, Eva said, "I'll go to the moon with you."

They got married in a massive thunderstorm and honeymooned in Italy. On September 26, the couple headed to the tiny Vienna airport and boarded a modified US bomber with four prop engines and makeshift seats for the long transatlantic flight. As they reached the shores of America, the red and yellow foliage of a New England fall spread out below them like a blanket of color welcoming them home.

CHAPTER ELEVEN

Alarm bells rang inside Presby. David Lawrence's heart—already brought back to life once and only with the effort of ten physicians—had stopped a second time. The sound sent nurses and doctors flooding back into the room for another attempt to save the dying ex-governor. Outside, politicians and reporters, all anxious for any news at all, paced the halls. Lawrence teetered so erratically between life and death that no news could be delivered even now, hours after he'd arrived at the hospital.

It was going to be a long night.

WHEN LAWRENCE FIRST collapsed at the Syria Mosque, Assistant Police Superintendent William Gilmore called Presbyterian-University Hospital with a heads-up that startled the staff into furious preparation. The ambulance arrived about fifteen minutes later. Three doctors and two nurses were there to meet them, with another dozen on the way. Safar rushed to the governor's side as his stretcher was pulled from the ambulance. He was surprised to see nurse Karen McGuire hop out of the back, but much less so to learn the cops had driven so recklessly she hadn't really been able to do anything. He did a quick assessment, found Lawrence to be "clinically but not biologically dead," and rushed him inside for treatment.

Fifteen staff members scrambled to start IVs, connect Lawrence to EKGs, and remove his clothes and jewelry. Emergency medicine wouldn't be recognized by the American Medical Association as a specialty until 1972, which meant there were no dedicated ER doctors. Safar was in charge. He sent up the order to begin CPR. The first step was to open the airway, done simply by tilting Lawrence's head as if he was sniffing something. Next was to provide two rescue breaths with a reusable ventilator. This was followed by chest compressions. A nurse placed two hands, one atop the other, over Lawrence's sternum and, bending at the waist, manually pumped his heart by forcibly compressing the chest wall. As they do with good CPR, Lawrence's ribs broke free from his sternum in a cascading series of pops like cracking knuckles.

By this point the cardiac monitor was ready, and an EKG showed his heart to be in ventricular fibrillation, a frantic, almost hysterical fluttering of the lower chambers. When this happens, no blood is being pumped, the heart's not even really beating, and the surest way to fix it is with electricity. Safar shocked him once—two charged paddles, one placed directly over the heart and the other midway up the left ribs—jolting Lawrence's body off the table and returning his pulse to normal. Next Safar prepared to intubate—he grabbed a laryngoscope, basically a tiny pickax, and used it to open Lawrence's mouth and pull his tongue out of the way, so the doctor could see down Lawrence's throat and past the white V of his vocal cords into his trachea. Safar slipped a breathing tube down, then connected it to the ventilator.

He was now breathing for the governor, and what he heard with each breath was a wet rumbling sound. This was troubling. Lawrence had vomit in his lungs, which causes pneumonia or a collapsed lung, and with a patient in so delicate a condition, those were complications Safar could not abide. He carefully suctioned Lawrence's last meal from his lungs, and the governor, who'd already regained his pulse, began breathing once again. By this point, he'd been in the hospital for twenty-five minutes.

Safar stood back to take stock. A patient who arrived clinically dead had been saved from biological death—*death* death—and was now critical but stabilized. There were tests to be run, of course, and Lawrence was still unconscious and unresponsive. Whether or not a seventy-seven-year-old man could plausibly survive what he'd just been through was very much an open question, but they'd made progress, and that Safar would take.

THAT WAS HOURS earlier. Now they were right back where they'd started, alarm bells ringing. Compressions and ventilations, medicine's synchronized hands working in fluid motion to perform the fickle art of resuscitation. This bout, the governor's second with death, lasted ten minutes. The third time his heart stopped, they would get it going in only five. By eleven p.m., Lawrence's pulse and breathing had once again been restored, and his blood pressure "was beginning to respond." But a fuller and more troubling picture began to emerge—Lawrence's brain was showing no signs of organized activity, calling into question whether he had any chance of recovery. This was a particularly hard development to swallow for Safar, who'd spent years trying to prevent this very thing from happening.

CHAPTER TWELVE

In 1956, the Safars were living in Maryland, where Peter was chief of anesthesiology at Baltimore City Hospital. He pursued his new field with a passion that bordered on obsession. He was so determined to improve the process of anesthesia that he tested the gases on himself. Cyclopropane, halothane, nitrous oxide, ether. He'd try anything, and if he liked the overall experience and the gas wasn't already being used at his hospital, he'd introduce it there himself.

Even when Safar wasn't working, he was working. Always plotting. And more and more of the plotting surrounded resuscitation. At that time, if someone stopped breathing for any reason—choking or drowning, an allergic reaction—the only treatment was an archaic sequence of steps known as the "back-pressure arm-lift" method. Essentially, this involved three phases: first, you rolled the victim facedown on the ground and straightened their arms out in a Superman position; next you knelt at their head and pressed once on their back, just below the shoulder blades; finally, you lifted and lowered their arms as if flapping the wings of a Thanksgiving turkey. You could repeat the process until something changed (nothing ever changed), but that was it.

It didn't sound as if it did anything, it didn't look as if it did anything, and as far as Safar could tell, it didn't in fact do anything. But people were still doing it. Lives were being lost every day, and yet nobody seemed to notice. Not the surgeon general, the Red Cross, the American Medical Association, no one. Safar was certain there was a better way, and in October 1956 he found the proof he'd been looking for.

The key to it all came from Dr. James Elam, a domineering physician from Texas. Atmospheric air—the air all around us—contains more oxygen than we use, and Elam proved that we not only breathe in but also breathe out this extra oxygen. His 1954 study showed we exhale so much extra oxygen that someone else could stay alive just by breathing in what we breathe out. In a world where the best-known method for saving someone who'd stopped breathing was to flap their arms (!), somehow for two whole years nobody had recognized the potential in Elam's findings. Safar saw it immediately.

The maverick physician from Vienna had long theorized that mouth-to-mouth could save lives. Now he was certain. To convince the rest of the world, he decided to stage a series of tests in which live volunteers would be sedated and paralyzed, then treated with both the old method and mouth-to-mouth to see which was better. It was a large and ambitious effort, and to pull it off Safar would need support, facilities, staff. He'd also need money. Baltimore was within striking distance of the nation's capital, close to a number of research universities, plus the National Research Council and the myriad medical organizations that fell under the umbrella of the National Institutes of Health. Obtaining funding for a project of this potential should have been easy. But everyone said no.

It's not hard to imagine, in 1956, what made Safar so untouchable. He was largely unknown, and what people did know, perhaps, wasn't entirely reassuring. He was only thirty-three. And he was a foreign-born physician with an unproven specialty. Not to mention the fact that he was trying to upend a hundred years of medical doctrine. No one believed in him, and so no one believed in his plan.

Getting spurned by the medical establishment raised more than just the specter of professional frustration. Safar had entered into this quest because he thought he was right, but more importantly he was doing it because he *had to*.

It wasn't long after the end of World War II before the full picture of what had happened—or at least its outline—became clear. The atrocities and destruction, the unspeakable loss of life brought by the Nazis not just on Austria but on the world was unimaginable. Safar had survived, his family too, but so many others had not. A third of his high school classmates were killed. Eighty percent of the kids who graduated the year before him never came home. The city was destroyed. Europe was in tatters. Some facts of the Holocaust would emerge all at once, others in a trickle over decades. It would be many years before Safar learned that some of the cadavers he and his classmates had dissected during the war were those of executed political prisoners.

Ignited by what later generations would call survivor's guilt, Safar vowed to push himself, would keep pushing himself well into his eighties, to almost inhuman levels, to return the gift of life that had been granted to him but denied to so many others. His survival was a heavy weight to bear and one he could manage only by returning the favor in-kind. If people were dying and he knew how to save them but didn't, then what was the sacrifice for? Why millions of others and not him? To prove himself worthy of having been saved, to repay the debt, he now had to prove he was right. And the tests were the only way to do that. Those were the stakes. If no one was with him, he'd go on alone.

Safar had never conducted a study of his own, and now he was staking his professional reputation on one he would develop, coordinate, staff, and fund all by himself. But he was too determined and idealistic to see the risks, and anyway, when the obstacles were obvious and insurmountable, he simply ignored them. For months he worked furiously in his free time to nail every detail. It all had to be perfect. And so did he. To prove mouth-to-mouth worked, he'd have to keep the sedated volunteers alive while also recording the physiological response to the *ways* he was keeping them alive. It was all about data. Empirical and undeniable evidence.

To capture it, each test subject would be attached to a series of monitors tracking—before, during, and after the tests—their heart rate, blood pressure, and oxygen levels, as well as how much or little the various methods of resuscitation inflated their lungs. All this was either explained to, or already understood by, the test subjects. So too did they have a working knowledge of Safar's cocktail of IV sedatives and paralytics, which included curare, the compound once used in the Amazon to make poison arrows. The sedatives, given first, rendered them unconscious. Once out, the victim would then be paralyzed, head to toe, unable to draw even the slightest breath. At this point they would be perilously (but safely) close to "clinical death" and entirely vulnerable, living proof of Safar's theory.

Whatever the risks, however unappealing it sounded to play a completely helpless human guinea pig, Safar had no trouble recruiting volunteers. Offered only $150 and a chance to make medical history, thirty-two doctors, nurses, and med students agreed to be rendered unconscious and unable to breathe for hours at a time. And they agreed to do this not once but repeatedly, over the course of forty-nine separate experiments. It signaled their dedication to medical advancement but also a tremendous amount of trust in a doctor who'd never done anything like this before.

And because the goal of his study was twofold—to prove one life-saving technique worked and also demonstrate that another didn't—he would have to subject his victims to a combination of both. First, they would be treated by medical professionals performing the back-pressure, arm-lift method. Next, they would receive the new mouth-to-mouth method that Safar had convinced them was superior. The second part wouldn't be performed by professionals, though. Instead, the one method that could, possibly, keep them alive would be administered by people who were untrained. Very untrained. To show just how easy to learn and effective mouth-to-mouth was, Safar recruited, among other laypeople, Boy Scouts as young as ten to keep his victims alive.

THE FIRST TEST was held on Saturday, December 8. For the location Safar chose one of the operating rooms at Baltimore City Hospital because they were closed on the weekend, so he and his odd assortment of volunteers would be left undisturbed. The OR was large and gleaming white, scrubbed sterile, and crammed with equipment and people. The victims were laid out on the floor, awaiting their fate. Standing around them, watching in an anxious semicircle, were the rescuers. Men in ties, women in dresses, all with hands clasped or arms folded, their faces full of grave concentration. Sprinkled throughout were the Boy Scouts. Buzz cuts and those perfectly folded scarves, uniform shirts bristling with the patches of past achievement. These children stood, hips cocked, as if they were ready, as if they'd always been ready. Eva, too, stood among this group of rescuers.

She had been there the day Peter learned about the study on exhaled air and had followed his line of thinking from inspiration to execution. She thought this was all quite daring, and though she'd never tried to resuscitate anyone or even witnessed mouth-to-mouth, she agreed to take part because she never once doubted that Peter had everything under control and that, if necessary, he could avert disaster. Besides, there was no room for doubt. Not with Peter. She would stop short of calling him arrogant, but only after acknowledging its possibility. She thought him young and entirely sure of himself, immune to the fear of failure.

Given that this was Safar's first demonstration and that he'd recruited untrained rescuers to carry it out, he could have been excused for keeping it quiet as a hedge against failure. Instead, he invited James Elam, the doctor whose study had provided the initial spark of inspiration. Elam was not entirely an ally and in fact had begun to feel his initiative was being stolen by this young upstart who'd turned his thoughts into action. He was veering from a spirit of friendly cooperation to one of fierce competition. If this demonstration didn't go well, if Safar's theory was disproven or his methods shaky, Elam had both the stature and the motivation to drive a stake into his heart. But he also had access to deep pockets of funding. For a man perfectly willing to bet on himself, this seemed to Safar a gamble worth taking.

Dressed in white scrubs, Safar began by sticking an IV needle into the arm of each of his victims. Once the line was running, he slowly pushed the sedatives. This took multiple doses and several minutes, but little by little, one heavy eyelid at a time, they all slipped into unconsciousness. Next came the paralytics, this stage going faster than the first, the deadly serious undertaking gathering a momentum of its own until the victims were fully paralyzed. They were now unconscious and not breathing, reliant solely on their rescuers, and would remain this way for three hours.

He started with the old method—back-pressure, arm-lift—which meant that his professional, Chief Martin McMahon from the Baltimore Fire Department, was up first. The simulated victims were now as close to actual victims as the healthy and willing can get. They weren't breathing and, if something wasn't done quickly, could go into cardiac arrest in only a few minutes. It would be impossible to overstate just how close to the edge Safar was pushing it at this point. Forget for a moment that they weren't breathing. Because the victims were unresponsive and their airways unprotected, if during the demonstration one of them vomited, they'd be unable to stop themselves from choking on it. Gone unnoticed or left uncorrected, it could kill them. And if it were to happen now and someone died, it wouldn't just be the end of the study but possibly the end of Safar's career.

Safar carefully disconnected the first victim's oxygen and the ventilator. Immediately his oxygen level began to drop. His blood pressure went up, and so did his heart rate, which only increased the demand for oxygen. Already, the body was screaming for air. With a nod, Safar moved out of the way and let McMahon begin. The chief rolled his victim over, placed him in the face-down, arms-out position, and begin trying to resuscitate him. Elam watched as the experienced firefighter expertly performed the old maneuver. It certainly looked like something had to be happening. But unlike in a real emergency, here the victim and the rescuer were both being measured by carefully calibrated machines. And what they showed was that, rather than pumping oxygen into the lungs, the procedure was actually squeezing it *out*.

Safar called a halt. He reoxygenated his victim, then turned to the untrained rescuers. They still didn't know what to do. To show mouth-to-mouth could be taught to, and performed by, anyone, Safar needed them to be as ignorant of the process as possible. Unlike the victims—who were told in excruciating, step-by-step detail precisely what would happen—the rescuers were intentionally left in the dark until the absolute last moment. He now explained in the briefest, most cursory terms what to do.

Then he stepped aside and waved a child forward. The weight and size disparity were striking. A two-hundred-pound man at the mercy of a seventy-pound boy. The Boy Scout knelt by the victim's head, tilted his chin up, and breathed. Nothing happened. The chest didn't rise, oxygen wasn't delivered. Maybe he had the wrong head position or hadn't closed off the nose or was simply not strong enough to force air into a full-grown man. No matter. With all the assurance of youth, he calmly readjusted, placed his mouth over the victim's, and breathed. This time, Safar and Elam watched as the chest rose, then fell and rose again, each breath delivering life to an unresponsive victim whose skin was already regaining its healthy flush of pink. Across the room, monitors showed the oxygen level was going up. The heart rate was slowing, the blood pressure lowering. It worked. Mouth-to-mouth, even performed by a child, worked. Each time, with every victim and all of the inexperienced volunteers, including Eva herself, the results were the same.

Elam was ecstatic. "We never dreamed the mechanical methods could be this bad," he told the press. Mouth-to-mouth, the technique inspired in part by his 1954 study, worked brilliantly, while the old methods "either moved no air or so little they were totally ineffective."

Safar, quiet in victory, concurred. "The old methods simply don't work. The victims can't get air."

He may not have been boastful, but he wasn't complacent. Safar conducted more tests, forty-eight more as planned, and he invited other influential figures to join him, including representatives of the American Red Cross—a group so taken with what they saw that they immediately spread the gospel to their colleagues in the International Red Cross. Elam was working with the Army Medical Research and Development Command out of Walter Reed Army Medical Center and ran straight to his military backers and convinced them to fund the effort. Safar, who just a few months before couldn't get a dime from anyone, now found himself flush with cash. Just as importantly, he'd soon have a way to preach his idea not just to the few but to the many.

A DOCUMENTARY, PRODUCED by the army and shot at Walter Reed, opens with Safar narrating in his nasal and precise accent: "The experimental study you are about to see is one of eighteen similar studies, during which we compared various methods of artificial respiration." Filming the experiments had been the military's idea, but it was Safar who understood its full potential to turn the tide. Getting people to save lives meant first convincing them they could. And however empirical the data might be, nothing compared to actually witnessing it. This film would make that possible. And because there were sure to be skeptics in the crowd, Safar decided to up the stakes.

During the live demonstrations, he minimized the time his victims went without oxygen. But now, for the filming of the movie, he did something different. With the camera trained on Dr. Felix Steichen—one of his sedated victims—Safar intentionally let Steichen's oxygen levels drop. Then he let them drop some more. And further still. He withheld oxygen until Steichen's levels dropped to 80 percent, a reading that would spur aggressive treatment by any emergency room in the country. The sight of a patient rapidly inching toward catastrophe created a dramatic moment that was only heightened when a Boy Scout stepped into frame with Steichen teetering on the edge, the boy knelt over him and with a few quick puffs of air rapidly brought him back from the brink.

It was yet another gamble that paid off. When the film was released, Safar barnstormed the country, drawing huge audiences. But it was the arresting sight of a child saving an unconscious adult that received breathless coverage in the press.

Nearly a year to the day after his initial inspiration, Safar flew to Los Angeles to formally present his findings. As he introduced to a panel of doctors the method of resuscitation that would ultimately save millions of lives around the world, the Soviet Union launched Sputnik into orbit—a chance confluence of events that marked October 1957 as both the dawn of the space age and also the birth of modern CPR.

By Safar's own recollection, the results landed like "a bombshell in the US and Europe." Global curiosity—about both CPR and the man who devised it—sent Peter and Eva on a whirlwind tour of Australia, New Zealand, Indonesia, Ceylon, Egypt, Lebanon, and Europe.

But even as people half a world away were embracing his ideas, he faced resistance at home. The data and the documentary were yawned at by the Maryland Medical Society, whose doctors were uninterested in any care—even if it was life-saving—delivered outside the hospital. And they balked at the idea of teaching medicine to the general public.

Plus, there was the elephant in the room.

At the very heart of Safar's innovation lay the unavoidable fact that for anyone to be saved by mouth-to-mouth, a rescuer must first place their mouth directly upon the victim's, which, often enough, would be the mouth of a stranger. To overcome this squeam-inducing prospect, Safar developed a small and inexpensive S-shaped device called the Resuscitube. This curved straw created a barrier between mouths. It was slightly less effective than direct ventilations but still provided enough air to keep someone alive.

If doctors didn't like Safar teaching medical procedures to laypeople, they liked even less that he was now teaching such people to use medical equipment. Following a demonstration in New Jersey, the chairman of the State First Aid Council insisted the tube would be too hard to use and feared "overzealous rescuers" would hurt people. Resistance emerged from all quarters. In its August 1959 issue, *Consumer Reports* magazine called the Resuscitube a "poor device for anyone to use," noting in particular that it should never be given to the "casual first aider." Though specifically disproven in the data, there were also lingering fears that victims would be poisoned during mouth-to-mouth by the rescuer's exhaled carbon dioxide.

Closer to home, Elam had been eclipsed by Safar's meteoric rise. Their relationship, which had begun on the razor's edge between cooperation and rivalry, now swung in the wrong direction. Safar found all of these "controversies, misunderstandings and jealousies" petty and emotionally draining. But he pressed on, overwhelming the opposition with the force of his personality and the pace of his innovation.

Even as hand-wringing continued over whether ordinary people could reliably and safely perform mouth-to-mouth, Safar pushed the issue even further by pairing it with chest compressions. For the first time, someone performing CPR was now not only breathing for the patient but also pumping their heart. This too took off around the world. In typically understated fashion, Safar named this super-charged version of CPR "Basic Life Support."

Call it what you want. For the first time in human history, someone who'd stopped breathing and had no pulse could be kept alive until they reached a doctor. CPR even preserved the health of the body's organs, including the one most likely to be damaged by a lack of oxygen—the brain.

CHAPTER THIRTEEN

Ten years after its invention, CPR performed by Karen McGuire didn't save Lawrence's life, but it kept him going, and in the days after his collapse, news of his condition—released in steady drips by his physicians—carried a note of befuddled optimism. For the moment, Lawrence was alive, which was cause for minor celebration, but the prognosis wasn't good. He was unconscious and unresponsive, heavily reliant on medical machinery, and given his age and all that he'd been through, he was expected to die at any time. But somehow he hung on. Pressed to explain it, Dr. Campbell Moses, Lawrence's personal physician, speculated that the governor simply refused to quit. "He's stubborn all over," Moses said.

What followed was a waiting game. For the governor and his doctors, even for the city's political elite. The gubernatorial candidate for whom Lawrence had been stumping, Milton Shapp, rushed to the hospital where he told reporters, "I will not return to the campaign trail unless I have assurance that Governor Lawrence will recover." Newspapers reported that Shapp—who would lose the following Tuesday to Republican Raymond Shafer—spent the night "stunned and grim-faced" in a conference room with Pittsburgh mayor Joseph Barr, Public Safety Commissioner David Craig, and a coterie of city and county officials.

But there would be no quick recovery, and the saga dragged on for weeks. The press kept a daily vigil. The doctors kept watch. The governor remained comatose.

Within hours of Lawrence's arrival at Presby, after his heart had been started and stopped then restarted again, Safar found little evidence of brain activity and surmised there simply was none. The following weeks did nothing to change his mind. So he and Moses sat down with Lawrence's family. The governor, he explained, was in a vegetative state and would not recover. The family decided to remove the governor from life support. Safar believed it was the first time such an action had been taken on a patient not "biologically dead." On the afternoon of November 21, 1966, seventeen days after he collapsed, David Lawrence "slipped away."

As the city mourned, Safar quietly fumed. Maybe there had been no avoiding it; maybe it was simply Lawrence's time to die. But maybe not. Help was there the night he collapsed. Karen McGuire—a medical professional—was doing CPR on him almost before he hit the ground, and Presby's doctors had his heart beating less than thirty minutes after he was brought in. Nevertheless, scans showed he had suffered severe brain damage. In the following days, he would occasionally blink but showed no other signs of life.

There was only one reason for this, and to Safar, it was as obvious as it was frustrating: poor ambulance care. A simple glance at the timeline showed that from the moment the police arrived at Lawrence's side until they dropped him off at Presby—just over ten minutes—he received no treatment, and his brain got no oxygen. The chain's only as strong as its weakest link, and here a criminally weak ambulance system had condemned an otherwise healthy man to die. Dr. Moses told the press that irreparable brain damage begins four minutes after the heart stops beating and that while efforts were made to save him, they weren't enough. "We've got to learn to do better in first aid," he said.

That a critical, life-saving network to provide emergency care in the streets would be called "first aid" shows just how far we were in 1966 from where we needed to be—and why it was so unlikely that we'd "do better." Still.

Street medicine, ambulance care, first aid—call it what you want. Dr. Moses was right: it was in a sorry state. For centuries, doctors and generals and politicians, public health experts of every stripe and qualification, had tried to make it legitimate. They'd gambled heavily on it, repeatedly, but the gamble rarely paid off and never for long. It didn't look or feel like traditional medicine and, despite their efforts, didn't conform to it. More and more the whole enterprise seemed hopeless. It was the racehorse with spirit but no pedigree, a feel-good story only until the end, because in the end it always lost.

But now, with the White Paper and the Highway Act, not to mention Safar's demonstration that medicine could be practiced on the fly by the uninitiated, there seemed to be the slightest glimmer of recognition that maybe, possibly, something should be done.

Still, the wise move for a physician, even one with Safar's wide-ranging ambitions, would've been to let someone else try to squeeze through the narrow opening created by Lawrence's death. It would take so long and consume so much. But Safar locked on. He was committed to the fight, driven by something other than his refusal to turn away from a challenge, something far more personal.

On the night of June 26, 1966, practically five months to the day before Lawrence collapsed, Peter and Eva were in Chicago for a meeting of the American Medical Association when they received a terrible phone call. Their oldest daughter, Elizabeth, at home with babysitters, had suffered a severe asthma attack and was on her way to the hospital. They rushed to the airport and caught the first flight back to Pittsburgh.

Elizabeth had been born premature nearly twelve years earlier and almost immediately showed signs of the struggle that would mark her life. Asthma had plagued three successive generations of Safars, including Peter's sister, Hanni, who would eventually die of asthma-related complications. But Elizabeth's was the worst case Peter had ever seen. From the time she was born, and nearly every night thereafter, her lungs had to be suctioned just so she could breathe. Her daily life was a stream of life-threatening crises combated by every treatment available, from home oxygen and aerosol inhalers—then a novel treatment—to a stay in a Swiss sanatorium. Nothing worked.

Elizabeth struggled so much that Safar would often rush home from work, usually dragging a respiratory therapist with him. Her attacks were frequent and severe. This one was different.

An asthma attack typically starts with tightness in the chest and a slight wheeze while breathing out. This is caused by a constriction of the airways, each exhaled breath whistling through narrowed passageways. It can be reversed with medicine, but in status asthmaticus—a persistent and rapidly worsening attack—a patient's lungs continue to constrict. As they shrink, the wheeze worsens. And it continues to worsen until there's no sound at all when the patient breathes out because they're not moving enough air to make any sound. It's now so difficult to draw a breath that their nostrils flare and the skin around their ribs sucks in with the effort. Confusion, exhaustion, anxiety, panic all quickly build as they get less and less air. They need more oxygen with every breath but each time are able to get less than the breath before. The spiral quickens and tightens, spinning out of control until they lose consciousness, and from there it's only a matter of time until they stop breathing altogether.

Safar arrived by Elizabeth's side at midnight. He found her not breathing and without a pulse. He immediately took over—imagine for a moment doing CPR on your own child—and, remarkably, was able to restart her heart and get her breathing. But that was it. He had come too late. She was and would remain comatose, her brain damaged from having gone too long without oxygen.

A week later, a little more than a month before her twelfth birthday, Elizabeth died.

Safar was an expert, perhaps *the expert*, on resuscitation and early intervention, and yet when his own daughter needed it, she could not be resuscitated because in her moment of need treatment did not begin early enough. To pile on the irony, Elizabeth's death came six years after firefighters in Baltimore, who Safar helped train in CPR, notched the first documented save of a patient in full cardiac arrest outside the hospital. It came five years after he began screaming that in an emergency, time is the enemy of the brain and that an emergency medical service—not hearses with drivers, but a *real* EMS, a fully integrated system that trained and equipped and dispatched qualified technicians directly to the scene—could get there fast enough and begin treatment early enough to preserve the brain so the patient could be saved. And it had been even less time since government officials first shot down his plans to launch such a system.

The man whose work had saved millions—the Father of CPR—had lost his oldest child to the very problem he'd been trying to solve. It was only when Pennsylvania lost a beloved governor months later that anyone else seemed to care. All he needed now was someone who could turn his thoughts into action.

CHAPTER FOURTEEN

At four minutes to three on the afternoon of November 21, 1966, a mechanic working on Big Ben dropped a ratchet into the old clock's winding mechanism, and, with a clatter, the whole thing ground to a halt. For twenty-two minutes that day, time in London stopped. Half a world away, as winter set in, the notoriously tough Steel City also paused, to remember the man it once knew as Mr. Democrat. The *Pittsburgh Press* reported that "Lawrence detested maudlin display and overstatement" and then promptly engaged in just that. Everyone joined in. Governor William Scranton, a Republican, ordered all the state's flags lowered to half-staff, and anyone whose name meant anything in the city came forward in a spirit of emotional eulogizing. State Supreme Court Justice Michael Musmanno: "Humanity has lost a great champion." US Senator Joseph Clark: "He leaves a record of achievement which will be difficult to equal." Farther afield, President Lyndon Johnson mourned "the passing . . . of a personal friend and trusted advisor."

In the Pittsburgh offices of the Maurice Faulk Medical Fund, morning papers spread out before him, Phil Hallen followed the news with growing interest. Hallen was middle-aged and slender, looking every bit the high school social studies teacher in his glasses and slowly thinning hair combed over just so, a collared shirt buttoned tight at his neck and cinched with a tie. Watching the attention attracted by Lawrence's death, Hallen recognized that a moment too long in coming was finally at hand.

Hallen arrived in Pittsburgh by a meandering, almost accidental, path. In 1952, he was working toward a PhD in English at Syracuse University and, like Safar before him and John Moon after, paying the bills with a part-time job as an operating room orderly at Crouse Irving Hospital. He carried bloody sheets, bandages, and patients—even their severed limbs—out of the OR and across the hospital, and it was on one such trip that Hallen saw a notice tacked to a bulletin board advertising an opening for attendants in the hospital's ambulance service. He had no particular interest in ambulances, had hardly even seen one, but he had a big interest in the free room and board given to anybody willing to drive one. So he applied.

For the next few years Hallen witnessed everything—birth to death—from the front seat of a beige, hearse-style ambulance. He had no idea what he was doing. But then neither did anyone else. Realizing how outmatched they were in serious emergencies, Hallen studied up on first aid as best he could and between this informal schooling and his experience on the job, he became better prepared for most emergencies than the brand-new doctors occasionally sent to assist him.

"Just stand back and look like you know what you're doing," he'd tell the new residents staring wide-eyed at the madness around them.

Hallen eventually dropped out of his doctoral program and enrolled instead in Yale's School of Public Health. In 1963, he moved to Pittsburgh and shortly after was named president of the Maurice Falk Medical Fund. The Fund was an offshoot of the much larger Falk Foundation, a noted and decades-old nonprofit named for the wealthy Pittsburgh family that ran it, titans of industry who among other things founded the company that became the National Steel Corporation. Not one to be lost in the shuffle, the scrappy Hallen quickly made the place his own. In the three years before his arrival, the Fund had given out just five grants worth $253,000. Over the next three years, under Hallen's guidance, it awarded fifty-eight, totaling nearly $2 million. He also established a system by which he could bypass the

Fund's bureaucracy to hand out $1,000 grants rapidly and solely at his own discretion.

Hallen's arrival coincided with the dawn of the civil rights era, and his mission was very much in step with the times. Asked to define the aim of the Fund, he once said, "What we are searching for is some method . . . of lessening the effects of bigotry and hatred." Specifically, the goal was to patch holes that systemic racism had cut into the public health safety net.

The poor state of ambulance care in his new city caught his eye early. Seeing Pittsburgh's police wagons, he told colleagues, "We're twenty-five years behind the times." In Pittsburgh, there were basically three systems. On the edges of town, ambulances were operated by funeral homes, so calls for help summoned a hearse operated by two undertakers who first had to sweep the flower petals from the back before responding to your emergency. If you lived farther out, on the edges of Allegheny County and beyond, your distress call reached a volunteer fire department. The people who manned these were unpaid and poorly trained. The firehouses had the atmosphere of a hangout, a sort of working man's country club resistant to change, particularly when it came to improving the training and equipping of their crews. When the topic came up, the response was always the same: Where would the money come from, and would the crews, volunteers after all, willingly take it? Either way, it rarely happened. In Pittsburgh proper, the job fell to the police, who, as evidenced by the circus atmosphere surrounding their attempted rescue of David Lawrence, often weren't trained or equipped to properly handle the job.

All this if you were lucky.

In the city's Black neighborhoods, service was worse. Ambulance cops didn't carry guns, but they often arrived with, and looked like, those who did. Relations between police and Pittsburgh's Black community were acrimonious at best, and people in the Hill didn't trust them. Calling the police for medical help could be a humiliating experience. They carried the same tone and demeanor with the sick as they did with the criminal. And that's if they showed up. Police regularly assumed a sick person in the Hill was really just a drunk person in the Hill and either mistreated or refused to transport them. Sometimes they skipped the call entirely.

Hallen harbored no illusions that he could start an emergency medical service, but maybe he could help build a network to take Hill District residents—a population with little access to health care—to and from the doctor's office. Since nothing even this simple existed, Hallen had to find someone willing and able to create it from scratch.

Here his idea took a radical direction. He knew from experience that successful community organizations couldn't be controlled from afar. They had to be staffed and operated, *had to be owned*, by the people they served. Working in the Hill, then, meant working with people of the Hill. It meant that this ambulance service, however modest in scope, had to be an entirely African American operation.

Much like Safar over at Presby, Hallen felt that he was the only one who recognized the ambulance problem staring them in the eye. But maybe David Lawrence's death changed that. Maybe now there'd be enough political will to get something done. Hallen decided it was worth a shot. But first he had to find someone who knew how to run an ambulance service.

By February 1967, Hallen had found what he was looking for—something called Freedom House Enterprises—but needed an introduction to set it up. He rushed over to City Hall and walked into the office of Moe Coleman, a staffer for Pittsburgh mayor Joseph Barr, and insisted, "I need to talk to Jim McCoy at Freedom House." Direct as ever. "Why don't you get us together?"

Freedom House was the brainchild of McCoy, a civil rights activist, with the long-term goal of fostering Black-owned businesses. In the meantime, to build capital as the organization got on its feet, Freedom House was selling produce in the street from the back of a truck. And it was this truck that grabbed Hallen's attention—if you could move produce, then you could probably also move people. At least that's how Hallen saw it.

Though it'd been decades since he left the steel mill and even longer since he'd worked in a brickyard, James McCoy Jr. still had powerful hands. Even at forty-eight and in a suit, he had the hands of a man put here to work. Born in Houston in 1919, McCoy was a preacher's son who was just seventeen when he moved, alone, to Pittsburgh. He started out in a brickyard but quickly landed a job at Continental Steel Rolling Foundries. Passionate about the plight of workers and gifted with a preacher's urgent and eloquent speech, he was elected president of Local 1904 of the United Steelworkers Union. Eventually McCoy left the mill to join Pittsburgh's civil rights community, rapidly rising in the local NAACP before founding the United Negro Protest Committee. He was twice arrested for demonstrating in the street and was among the delegates selected to receive Martin Luther King when he came to town in 1966.

McCoy was no longer a young man, but he still had the fire of a man half his age, and he had recently started to feel hemmed in and slowed down by the protest community's older, stuffier leadership. He wanted the freedom to make decisions and take action. So in January 1967, he started an organization of his own and named it Freedom House Enterprises in honor of breaking loose. Its headquarters was a tiny storefront in the Hill, squeezed next to a clothing store, with several floors of crowded apartments above them. As Hallen passed through the door, papered over with advertisements for an upcoming voter registration drive, and walked beneath the words *FREEDOM HOUSE* painted in giant block letters, it would've been hard to miss the energy or to think he was anywhere but the right place.

Phil and Jim were more or less opposites. Hallen was white and from the northeast, practical and to the point but also an improviser. McCoy, a Black man from the South, spoke leisurely and philosophically, his thoughts strung together by looping sentences that hid within them evidence of his immovable convictions. Asked why he'd left a union job to join the civil rights movement, McCoy said, "A person does not get into the movement. The movement is in a person."

At their first meeting, however, it was Hallen who did the talking. And the plan he'd come to discuss didn't sound practical to McCoy. In fact, it was significantly more ambitious and far-reaching than anything Freedom House was doing or might conceivably be able to pull off at this point. The organization's goals in those early days were fairly modest, and its nascent jobs program was focused mainly on training Hill residents for domestic or maintenance work. This gradual rise to critical mass was in keeping with McCoy's philosophy of patient but persistent resistance, typified by a rhyme he often shared: "little drops of water / little grains of sand / make a mighty ocean / and a pleasant land."

Hallen blew right by this measured approach. His idea wasn't to train people in landscaping. He wanted to turn them into health care providers, giving Black people in the Hill precisely the sort of thing John Moon found so incredibly elusive: a coveted entrée into the field of medicine. They would also need people for logistics, mechanics to work on the trucks, and the whole thing, from providers to support staff to equipment—all of it—would be owned and operated by locals. Hallen's vision covered the whole spectrum of training, employment, and enterprise. Nothing like it existed. It was revolutionary even before taking into account that it would give residents of the Hill District, for the first time, ready and easy access to health care.

This was more than drops of water and grains of sand, more than Freedom House was ready to handle. But then McCoy had been in the movement—or rather it had been in him—for over a decade. He'd seen how hard the work was, how stiff the resistance. He'd spent time in jail, and even a year before Dr. King's death he knew what potentially could be on the horizon. What had happened in Watts and Newark and Harlem, in Detroit, the riots and looting, the fires—he'd been around a long time and had participated in enough demonstrations to know that, even if the Hill had never seen violence, people were angry and desperate and eventually the cap would fly off.

The only way to avoid that would be to offer African Americans in Pittsburgh a path out of poverty. A real one. Opportunities beyond housecleaning or lawn cutting. And Hallen was proposing a chance to do just that. Backed by a foundation with the ability to provide quick infusions of cash, Freedom House could offer more than just menial jobs and manual labor; it could provide something to make things better, to make real change.

McCoy held out a powerful hand to Hallen. He was in.

CHAPTER FIFTEEN

"Go talk to Safar." This was practically the first thing Hallen and McCoy heard when they began asking around about an ambulance service. Millions of dollars in Falk Medical Fund grants circulated through the Pitt School of Medicine, so Hallen was familiar with Safar. He knew all the Father of CPR stuff and knew also how the Austrian doctor had, with his wife, Eva, so thoroughly dominated the city's annual waltzing contest that in decency and fairness they permanently retired from competition. But none of this gave him any real indication of what Safar's interest in ambulances might be. Frankly, Hallen wasn't entirely clear on his own ideas for creating an ambulance service. What he had, really, was the piece of an idea, and as he and McCoy entered Safar's office, they quickly began to realize just how small a piece of the bigger idea it actually was.

Safar had already tried (and failed) to start an ambulance service in Pittsburgh. He'd brought with him from Baltimore plans for a comprehensive EMS system but ran into resistance from doctors and the police department brass, and though he continued to agitate for change, his efforts were mired in political infighting. Besides, people were used to the police wagons and the hearses and either didn't think there was a problem or, if they did, kept those feelings to themselves. Either way, nobody had any interest in improving the situation. Safar did, of course, but he didn't do small or modest, and though he saw the glint of possibility within the Freedom House proposal, he wasn't interested. There was an opportunity here to do something truly remarkable, but to get him on board they'd have to think bigger, grander. They'd have to rewrite the rules.

Safar told Hallen and McCoy that the prevailing ambulance theory of rushing patients to the hospital was backward and ought to be dumped on its head. What they needed instead was an entirely new model of ambulance work: he wanted to bring the emergency room to the patient and begin treatment right there on the pavement. This had been tried in shades, like the doctors on New York's nineteenth-century ambulances, but nothing quite so revolutionary. The system couldn't and wouldn't rely on doctors or barely trained cops. Instead, he wanted to train paramedics—a phrase just then coming into existence—in a wide range of medical and traumatic emergencies, and give them a wider scope of practice than any of their predecessors. They should be able to deliver babies and handle hemorrhages and open fractures, cardiac arrests, spinal injuries. They should know how to suction respiratory patients, he said, then took it a step further and insisted they also learn to intubate—a technique that, in 1967, only doctors could perform. Of course, to really be effective, medics would need to give IV fluids and a whole cabinet of medications. So, while they were at it, why not teach them how to start IVs? He believed all this to be not only vital but possible, achievable in the near term even in a city whose existing ambulance attendants had never heard of CPR.

He'd also given extensive thought to the ambulance itself. Safar felt the patient compartment must be redesigned so care could start fast and continue all the way to the hospital. It would need to provide room for two medics to work simultaneously, providing uninterrupted CPR and airway control in a moving vehicle. No more patients flopping lifelessly and alone in the back of a police wagon. Not one more salvaged body functioning at the behest of an unsalvageable brain.

Safar wanted to end the "swoop and scoop" process that typified ambulance work, in the process changing an entire culture. And as the guy who'd recently defied and reshaped the practice of medicine probably more than any other doctor, Hallen and McCoy believed he could pull it off. Without realizing it, certainly without meaning to, they had stepped into the middle of a revolution.

As for what role they could play, Safar already had that part nailed down too. Tireless as he was, always plotting, even he needed help transforming his ideas into action and what he needed more than anything was manpower. And the critical piece missing from his plan had just walked quite unexpectedly through his door.

"I've been trying to figure out how to take these ideas," he said, "these scientific experiments . . . out to the street. You're exactly what I'm looking for."

Hallen was astonished. No such thing as Safar was now proposing existed. As far as he knew, no one had even thought of it. There was no established training, no awareness, no field of study. Nothing. Nationwide, the entire ambulance industry was so slapdash and chaotic—the job itself so poorly defined and performed there wasn't even a name for the people who did it—that only years later would regular Americans look back on this time in shock and wonder aloud, *What the hell was going on?*

Hallen shot a look at McCoy. "So . . . we can certainly do that but—"

But.

Everything hung in that *but*. It was the nexus of the very problem, of so many problems. What Safar was proposing, it all sounded great, but it also sounded technical and advanced, requiring expertise, which wasn't just one thing but *the* thing that had brought Hallen and McCoy together. The Black community, particularly those living in the Hill, had no access to much of anything technical or advanced or requiring expertise. And so . . . but—

Safar waved them off.

"I'm trying to train people, who don't have the slightest bit of training, to be professionals," he said.

Here once again was the maverick side of Safar's energy and genius. He didn't simply want to prove that an advanced form of medicine could be practiced in the street. He wanted to show it could be copied in duplicate, triplicate—a thousand times over in a thousand other cities—and to do that he'd first have to demonstrate that regular people with no medical training could be turned into professionals. You weren't going to get doctors and nurses to do this job. A century of fits and starts had already shown that. You had to create something new, something affordable, something that'd been designed for this rather specific and peculiar purpose. To create the work, in other words, you first had to create the worker. The paramedic.

"I want ordinary people," Safar said. "It sounds like you've got a lot of ordinary people."

Hallen and McCoy were right there with him. "Oh, we have ordinary people. High school dropouts and all the rest."

In no way was this the plan they'd come here to push, but Hallen and McCoy understood that grassroots community organizing was jazz, unstructured and free, and so they were prepared to follow a good idea wherever it led. Were they in? Of course they were in. Hallen crowed: "You've got the gas; we've got the bus!"

For Hallen and McCoy, there was only one point on which there could be no improvising or deviation, where the music had to be played, every note, just as it was written. These ordinary people Safar would train to do extraordinary things, they would all be Black.

They knew there was the potential for pushback on this issue, that if Freedom House faced overt opposition, whether from the start or later on down the road, it would be over the question of race. Nevertheless, more than an innovative jobs program or a revolution in emergency medicine—and it was definitely both of those things—the Freedom House ambulance corps was to be first and foremost a beacon of pride. In a place like the Hill District, where the world took a whole hell of a lot without ever giving back, where crime and poverty were at all-time highs, where people were referred to as "unemployables," the sight of a young Black man stepping from an ambulance in service of his community would restore a measure of dignity even to those who witnessed it. And as he blazed a trail for others to follow, that medic's achievements would reach far beyond the Hill, helping to stamp out the racist notion that it was a lack of ability—not inequality—that held African Americans back. Hallen and McCoy believed all this because they knew that the medics would be saviors to many thousands beyond the Hill who would never call on them for help.

If they ever worried the foreign-born Safar wouldn't understand, they needn't have. Here was a man who entered adulthood trapped in Nazi-occupied Austria, who witnessed, at a close remove, the Holocaust, and who embraced the progressive ethos of the '60s. He didn't blink. It was decided: the anesthesiology department Safar ran at Presby would provide Freedom House with the ambulances and the training that would turn their ordinary people into paramedics. Whom Hallen and McCoy chose to take that course would be left entirely to their discretion.

And just like that, in only thirty minutes, plans were set in motion for the world's first paramedic training class. The only question that remained was whether this mismatched group could pull off a feat that had thus far defeated all comers.

CHAPTER SIXTEEN

The larger world might've been skeptical of what they were trying to do, but those on the inside never doubted it. They were on the right side of history; they had momentum and conviction; they had the minds. Lord knows they had the experience. Aside from Safar and McCoy and Hallen, who carried with them the full weight of the University of Pittsburgh, Freedom House, and the Falk Medical Fund, they also recruited several energetic doctors from Safar's anesthesiology department, enlisted the Allegheny County Medical Society, included officials from the police department, and were assisted by key players from the staff of Mayor Joseph Barr, including Moe Coleman, whose role in the administration was to win Pittsburgh its share of the federal grants offered by President Lyndon Johnson's Great Society. On April 15, 1967—just three months after Hallen's *aha* moment with the produce truck—this klatch of heavyweights gathered for the first time.

The first item on the docket was money. The lightning-quick grants Hallen had the power to approve were small. They needed big money. In ordinary times, with no obvious analog to point to and say, "We're looking to do something just like that," a project this ambitious might scare donors off. But these weren't ordinary times. Thanks to President Johnson and the civil rights movement, the Kerner Commission, and shifting mores—sexdrugsandrocknroll, *Age of Aquarius!*—the country was changing. Or at least change was being considered, and among those considering it were the people in charge. One major initiative after another came down the pike from both the public and the private sectors. The War on Poverty, AmeriCorps, the Opportunities Industrialization Center, the Ford Foundation. The federal government alone was launching so many urban relief and renewal initiatives that in 1966 it created a program called Model Cities just to streamline the bureaucracy that'd sprung up around them. In the spring of '67, a million sources of funding and its attendant infrastructure—much of it designed specifically for Black communities—had been conjured up and let loose upon the world, and Freedom House, which touched every base, was poised to benefit from them all.

If they were optimistic about the prospect of funding, they were equally expansive in their vision for how it would be spent. About the ideal class size, Coleman, the resident grant wizard, asked, "How big? What are we talking here?" Safar said he could teach forty-four at a time. Forty-four. Dozens of people with zero medical experience and whose formal education might be a question mark winding their way through a yet-to-be-determined, first-of-its-kind course that had to prepare them—in three months? six months? twelve?—to hit the streets capable of assuming the awesome responsibility of saving human lives.

Seemed reasonable.

"Okay," said Coleman, scribbling on a pad. "Let's write a federal grant for whatever that'll cost and start off with a class of forty-four people."

So it went. Then they needed a base of operations, a place from which to launch these guys into disasters big and small. What fit the bill? Put them right in the Presby ER, close to the action, a physical link to the chain of care they'd help lengthen. Of course, their unique and irreplaceable role in that chain was mobility, and for that they'd need wheels. The Freedom House vegetable truck wouldn't do. A state-of-the-art paramedic service needed an ambulance to match. A grant proposal for a fleet of Freedom House ambulances was drawn up and sent out. It carried within its pages grand ambitions.

Envisioned in those early full-steam-ahead planning sessions was a fleet of ambulances, each with varying capabilities, comprising a kind of pyramid of engine-born readiness. On the bottom there would be a wheelchair ambulance for nonemergency transfers from one hospital to another, a decidedly unsexy task that nonetheless paid so well everyone was able to hold their nose and swallow it. Next, there'd be traditional ambulances to handle run-of-the-mill emergencies—a fall, an assault, dizziness, maybe the occasional drunk. And then there was the tip of the pyramid: a deluxe resuscitation ambulance bearing every design element, and all the equipment, that Safar could dream up. Carrying a physician if one was there to be conscripted at a moment's notice. The deluxe rig would be for the major emergencies—Governor Lawrence, Safar's daughter. High-stakes, life-and-death emergencies. The kind where you'd be handed the unspooling thread of someone's father, wife, or child, and either win big or lose it all.

In those weekly planning sessions, dreams were conjured, expanded, and combined. They were also, methodically and one at a time, dashed. Support from the county medical society, a little shaky from the start, evaporated. The cops were next, realizing a shade too late that Freedom House would eliminate not only the brand of negligent care delivered in their wagons but the jobs of those providing it as well. Then there was the money, which was coming but slowly—way too slowly, so slowly that they'd have to start without ambulances and instead use a pair of donated police wagons, repainted with the Freedom House logo, to act as stand-ins until the real thing arrived.

By October, Safar had grown impatient. There was optimism and hope and incredible ambition, but it was taking too long. One evening, he picked up the phone and started dialing. Over at Freedom House, Jerry Esposito answered. Esposito was a jack of all trades and something of an ambulance savant. Before joining Freedom House, he ran an ambulance service out of his kitchen: calls for help went directly to his house and were handled in the back of a Chevy Impala station wagon outfitted with lights and a handmade sign that read, "AMBULANCE." Over the phone, Safar told him the time had come. No more delays or doubts, no more waiting. His paramedic course would start in the morning.

This set off panic on Centre Avenue. Recruiting had been handled by an outside source, and it wasn't going well at all. Say what you want about adventure, about life and death, the chance to be a hero, the fact was they were asking people to sign up for a three-hundred-hour, eight-month training course to prepare them for a job that technically didn't exist. The whole thing was so unappealing—even in a neighborhood with a 14 percent unemployment rate—that they weren't even close to the forty-four students Safar had asked for back in April.

At Freedom House with Esposito that night were two other staffers. John Conley—young, blind, outspoken, an attorney instantly recognizable for his thick mustache and dark wayfarer sunglasses. Thelma Lovette—born the fifth of eleven children, lifelong civil rights activist with too many advanced degrees to count. They too were versatile outsiders, exactly the kind of brilliantly energetic people, unphased by long hours and impossible odds, that all unorthodox ideas need to survive. The three of them sprang into action.

Esposito drove the Hill in his Chevy Impala, promising free dinner to anyone who followed him back to Freedom House. John and Thelma walked up and down Centre, literally dragging people off the street. Together they roped in anybody not fast enough to get away.

And it worked. They made their quota. The great crusade was underway.

CHAPTER SEVENTEEN

In the morning, when Safar showed up to begin the course, forty-four men stared back at him from their seats. They were tired and not at all certain what they'd just signed on for. They were here for a common purpose, but each man had his own story. Arthur Davis, twenty-four, had dropped out of high school in the eleventh grade. Asked why, he said, "I have one of those funny minds. I just didn't take to math and English. It was hard to catch on." He'd been working ever since as an itinerant laborer. Dishwasher, garbage man, maintenance. He spent five months in Detroit at a dye-casting and spray paint company but was laid off and drifted back home. He was living with his mother.

Dave Rayzer was married with two children. He graduated high school in '62, spent a few years working as a bookbinder at Carnegie Library, but switched to manufacturing when his second child came along. That job, though better paying, lasted only a few months, and he was looking for something new when John Conley and Thelma came along.

They were men who existed on the margins and were looking for a way to get ahead, gambling on a long shot. Their ages ranged from eighteen to sixty. Nearly half hadn't completed high school. One had just a sixth-grade education. Some bounced from job to job, and others hadn't worked at all. A few had been to Vietnam and returned struggling with drugs and alcohol. Others had been urged to sign up by their mothers and grandmothers. Several had been convicted of violent crimes, like twenty-year-old Michael Blackman, who was arrested in December 1963 for a botched car theft and stabbing.

Conley felt the men he'd helped pull in off the street "had little to look forward to" before Freedom House, but he believed the program would transform them from "life-failures to life-givers."

Hallen was more anxious. He knew all the talk about respectable jobs, racing around in ambulances, saving lives—not to mention the higher goals of the program—had to be backed up with people who had the ability and courage to shepherd these men through what promised to be a very difficult course. Whether they pulled this off or fell flat on their faces depended almost entirely on Safar's ability to connect with his students and lead them through to the end. This was no small question. For all of Safar's big ideas and genius and drive, his ambition as a scientist and clinician, the one thing he definitely lacked was street cred.

Unlike the men seated before him, it was incredibly unlikely that Safar would ever be swept up in a casual canvassing of the Hill. He lived outside the city, in a four-bedroom colonial in the affluent suburb of Mount Lebanon. There, on a leafy street, he and Eva were raising a family and hosting their own version of a Viennese salon. Each month Safar, an accomplished pianist, would sit at his 1919 Bösendorfer baby grand and play for a rotating cast of foreign students, research fellows, doctors, and musicians. They hosted up to a hundred people at a time; many brought their own instruments or wrote a piece of music, while others danced or sat back and soaked it all in. For the artistic, the cultured, or simply the homesick, a night at the Safars' was a respite. Whether he would relate to these men or they to him was very much an open question.

The task before each of them—teacher and student alike—was enormous. The course would begin with fifty hours of instruction in anatomy and physiology. Students would then take CPR, advanced first aid, defensive driving, the fundamentals of nursing, and medical ethics and legalities. They'd learn how to recognize and treat cardiac arrhythmias, start IVs, and also handle and administer drugs. They'd learn how to deal with diabetic emergencies, arterial bleeds and compound fractures, hypothermia. Hyp*er*thermia. How to stabilize spinal fractures and pelvic fractures, overdoses, those with difficulty breathing and those who couldn't breathe at all. It would be an intense program of study, what one historian has called "exponentially more training than any non-physician civilian ambulance crew ever obtained."

From the beginning it was clear their new life wouldn't be an easy one. Before class even started, the students were shuttled through a bruising initiation. Psychological evaluations and personality tests. In-depth interviews with therapists. "Serial interrogations" with the hospital's medical staff and then again with the personnel department. This was not a rubber stamp. It was a gauntlet. By the time the process was over, the students Thelma and John and Jerry had worked so frantically to recruit just days before now saw their numbers whittled down from forty-four to twenty-five.

More attrition was yet to come. The schedule and pace of training made the endeavor especially demanding. Students struggled with IV insertion and—that classic American foil—learning the metric system. Techniques and terminology, medical shorthand, were all heaped on them. The men were forced to surrender not only their days but also nights and weekends to a grinding course that dragged on week after week. Tired and frustrated, students tunneling ever deeper into the complicated minutia of biology repeatedly called out, "Why do we need to know this?"

It took a toll. Ten students quit in the first three months. Others were kicked out for disciplinary issues. The twelve men who hadn't graduated from high school were also required to take a full slate of GED classes hosted by the city's public school system. Everyone felt bogged down and overwhelmed, and it soon became clear that what was intended to be an eight-month course would stretch into nine.

Seated in schoolhouse-style wooden chairs attached to desks, dressed in white button-down shirts and pants (sometimes with a black tie), the remaining students plowed on. Safar rooted the esoteric in the practical—*you're learning* that *because someday you'll have to do* this. Students dissected animals, trained on mannikins, studied X-rays and tissue samples from a slaughterhouse, and underwent an intense EKG rotation. Eight hours a day they stared at a wall of cardiac monitors, each screen displaying an individual patient's heart rhythm. Every blip gave a clue as to what was or wasn't happening with a given patient's heart. Learn to read EKGs, and you can diagnose the myriad things liable to go wrong with a heart—heart failure, heart attack, heart block, a heart that's beating too fast or too slow or not at all—and you'll know how to fix it. They'd also have to know how to use everything that would sit in a sealed drug box in the back of every Freedom House ambulance, a rainbow of pharmaceuticals (cardiac and otherwise). And from his seat at the patient's head—the seat Safar had specifically placed there—a medic would assess, diagnose, and treat all without ever setting foot in the hospital.

Lessons were drilled into their heads. Simplicity through repetition. The edges were sharpened, techniques honed to perfection. Finally, in early 1968 they completed the classroom portion of their training. The reward for making it this far? More hardship.

The twenty-four remaining students now began 172 hours of clinical training. They'd spend a week at the morgue assisting the coroner with autopsies, two weeks in the OR learning how to intubate from anesthesiologists, and another week in the ER. Only after they'd completed all this would they step foot in the streets, not their own but Baltimore's, where Safar had long-standing ties with the fire department that stretched back to the CPR study.

The idea of sending students directly from the classroom to the bedside where under supervision they could perform the skills they'd just learned, perhaps not coincidentally, mirrored the experience of medical school. Like that of other medical professionals, their training was all geared toward injecting the students into the hospital and making them an interlocking part of the system rather than an ancillary piece. They'd spend time in the OB ward because someday they'd be delivering babies on the side of the road. They went to the morgue to actually *see* the liver and aorta and the kidneys, put the whole complex thing together in their minds by first taking it apart with their hands. They went to the OR to practice intubation and the ER for everything else. Each step was a small piece of the larger whole the medics would be taking with them out into the street. If they went far deeper in class than they could possibly be expected to go in the street, then they'd be able, when disaster struck, to go wherever the situation required. So when they spent time with orthopedists, it was because someday, who knew when, somebody would get hit by a car, and their shattered femur would slice through muscle and skin, and the medics wouldn't panic because they'd have seen it firsthand and know just what to do.

Safar wasn't just training his students in medicine. He was baptizing them in it as well.

But unlike the classroom portion of their training, they couldn't practice medicine in a vacuum. They'd have to go out into the real world, lay hands on real people, and it was outside the safe confines of Safar's classes that the students got their first taste of the challenges that lay ahead. Despite the patches on their arms that read *Ambulance Attendant Trainee*, nurses startled by the sight of Black men approaching the OB ward refused them entry. It quickly became a whole scene, and Safar, called from his office, rushed down. Maybe he took the stairs two at a time thinking this was all just a misunderstanding. Probably the students themselves weren't surprised.

When Safar reached the OB floor, he tried to intervene, but the nurses were so insistent that his students ended up learning how to deliver babies from watching training films. The ER was another story. Students had spent months preparing to treat patients and arrived eager to begin the real work of practicing medicine. Instead, the nurses they were here to shadow simply assumed they were orderlies and handed them mops. It was the same thing happening all across the city, at steel mills and construction sites, where Black men were hired but not promoted, locked into menial roles—all the barriers and slights that were, at that very moment, driving John Moon to activism and his worried parents to distraction.

The indignities, one piled atop the other. But again the students pushed through, as they had all along, somehow keeping their composure, learning, training, getting closer. The mop might still be there in the corner, a reminder, but their eyes all the while remained on the finish line.

Yet the end point they were all so intensely focused on lay on the far side of Safar's most ambitious goal: intubation.

"You have thirty seconds to intubate this patient. Go."

That's how it started. The most intimidating thing the students would do throughout their training, arguably the most critical hands down the easiest to mess up—began with a ticking clock. Intubating is hard. Arthur Davis hadn't made it through high school, and now he was standing at the head of a surgical bed. An unconscious patient sprawled out before him, Peter Safar waiting behind him. Davis would have to peer through the narrowing tunnel of soft tissue leading from the patient's lips toward the twin openings at the back of her mouth. One led to the esophagus, the other to the trachea. Force the tube into the wrong one, and air would go to her stomach instead of her lungs, and the patient would die. This is easy to do. It's dark back there and hard to tell one from another. Plus the wrong one (naturally) is larger and easier to hit. He had to take his time but not too much. Too long, and the patient becomes dangerously short of oxygen.

This was live-fire training at its worst. He was only practicing, sure, but on a *real live person*. A woman who'd come in for routine surgery and now needed him to intubate her so she could get oxygen. Screw this up, and he would kill her. Twenty seconds to go. Ron Ragin, still trying to intubate, began to sweat.

Safar checking his watch, the monitors. Impatient. The pressure of the moment, the likelihood of failure, it was immense. *Fifteen seconds*. All eyes on Clyde Dunson. The tube began to feel enormous, the opening to the trachea impossibly narrow. *Eight seconds.* John Franklin squinting, trying to see. *Tick tick tick*. Ray Pridgen reached in with the tube and—"Time! Step aside please."

Safar moved the student to the side. It could be any of them; it went this way for everybody—Davis or Ragin or Dunson, for Franklin and Pridgen and also for Harvey Gandy, William Holland, William Porter, David Clemens, Dave Rayzer. They all struggled. And when they failed to get it done in time, Safar would take the endotracheal tube and do it himself.

Intubation training took a turn Safar hadn't foreseen and didn't have the time to adjust for. That the medics would master intubation had been the biggest question mark (perfecting the technique takes more time than they had) but also one of Safar's highest priorities. He was an anesthesiologist and specialized in airway management. An open and clear airway is the starting point, the baseline, of patient care. It's about whether or not a patient can breathe, and as the medical maxim goes, if you don't have an airway you don't have a patient. There was perhaps another side to it, though. The part that had to do with being the father of a child who died from an asthma attack, whose airways had slammed shut, and for whom the ride to a doctor who could intubate had taken too long. Maybe if a properly trained paramedic—maybe one of his own, who knows—had been there that day, well, maybe things would've turned out differently.

And so, despite the immense difficulties, the added strain on a course that was already pushed to its limits and running behind schedule, Safar persisted. He tried to convince other anesthesiologists to allow the students to practice on their patients. They all said no. He switched gears, tried to convince the morgue to let them practice, to convince funeral homes to let them practice. Every time it was the same answer. No. Not here. No way. He was limited to his own patients, and there weren't enough of those, not enough for every student to get the amount of practice he needed.

Reluctantly, Safar moved on. He vowed to come back to it, but for now he was forced to drop intubation from the list of skills the medics would master during their course. It was the first failure, and given the drive behind it, the stakes, for Safar it was a bitter one. For the men, it may have been a disappointment, but it was only one thing they hadn't learned as they approached the end of their training having learned so much.

At the end of the course, the students were to take a series of written and practical exams. Each needed a perfect score to graduate, and these were difficult tests. It would take some students two full weeks to get there. But before any of that, there was one more component of training to complete. Safar brought the class to Baltimore, where he'd worked out a deal with his old contacts at the fire department for his students to ride the ambulances. He wanted them to run real calls. To lay hands on actual patients. They arrived with more knowledge but less experience than the firefighters they were paired with, and this experience was meant to remedy that.

They never got the chance. April 4 came, and Walter Cronkite said, "Good evening," from the set of *CBS Evening News*, and Robert Kennedy said, "I have some very sad news," from a flatbed truck in Indianapolis, and a young man said, "Let's burn the damn place down," from the Hill.

They rushed back to Pittsburgh, where grief over Dr. King's assassination had turned to violence. The Hill was in trouble. No one was getting medical aid, so Freedom House commandeered a handful of police vehicles and drove the streets, interior lights turned on so people outside would see them and not shoot. They weren't yet done with their training, weren't yet making the $2.50 an hour they'd make as official paramedics, but still they showed up. While their neighborhood erupted, these men suited up and hit the streets.

They understood the anger and hurt and need to scream for the world to stop and take notice. They'd been raised in the Hill, had seen their home cut off and left for dead. They'd been ignored, made to feel they had no value, that they were powerless and voiceless. And so they'd put their lives on hold, surrendered to Safar's schedule and demands. They sweated through months of intense schooling. Grown men with children of their own kept their mouths shut in the smug face of indignity—*take this mop*—because from the very beginning, before they even knew what a paramedic was, they understood instinctively it was something the world could not ignore.

In this uniform, with that patch, they would be heard.

CHAPTER EIGHTEEN

In the small, crowded Freedom House base station just a few feet from the entrance to the Presbyterian-University ER, a phone rang. It was a rotary dial, black originally but later replaced by a red one. This was the hotline, and when it rang, Ruth Gardner—one of the dispatchers, all women, who would play a critical role in the success of Freedom House—stopped what she was doing to snatch the receiver. Ruth was young, hair pulled up in a shorter version of what the Ronettes might wear. She listened and started scribbling on a notepad. In Pittsburgh, calls for help went first to the city's Public Safety Building, and anyone requesting an ambulance in the Hill or Oakland or downtown was passed along to Freedom House. Ruth wrote down the particulars—address and nature of the emergency; whether the patient was stable, critical, or already dead—and then hung up. She passed the call to Dave Rayzer and Leroy Morant, who stood up, their third time in an hour, and rushed out.

The automatic doors swung shut behind Rayzer and Morant as they stepped out into the night. Rayzer was twenty-four with two kids and had graduated from Fifth Avenue High. Former bookbinder, former laborer. Formerly laid-off. A round welcoming face with a pair of eyeglasses. When the training program wrapped back in June, he finished at the top of the class, but that mattered less now than his ability to use all that information—and he'd already begun to show it—to treat the sick and injured, to control a crowd on the scene. He moved with casual grace toward the ambulance. His partner, Morant, was wire-thin with hair shaved close to the skin and all the way up the sides like a mohawk. In they went. Turn the key, press the gas. The engine rumbled to life.

When they arrived, their patient was unconscious on the floor. Another Oakland overdose. Maybe breathing, maybe not. Rayzer didn't need the associate degree in sociology he was working toward to explain why they were here or what had led this young man to desperate straits. He was a native son and needed only look out the window to see the wood and glass still in the street from April, block after block obliterated, never repaired. A neighborhood left broken, demoralized. And so was their patient. They got right to work.

An overdose is one of those peculiar emergencies, at once desperate and pedestrian. A killer that can, in the right hands, be easily killed himself. It's identified as often by the things that aren't there as those that are. Like a patient found living in a house that's not a home—no furniture or clothes, nothing at all that says someone lives here. Probably the man at their feet was turning gray all over. He definitely wasn't breathing. They repositioned his head, which was bent so far back he was blocking his own airway. Kneeling now, they ripped equipment from its packaging. Maybe they couldn't intubate—not yet—but they could still breathe for this man.

A deep puff of oxygen from the portable ventilator, fingers gripping the limp jaw to keep a good seal. Here it was all about technique. Do it wrong, and up comes a hot geyser of stomach water. They'd practiced this a thousand times under the particular and suspicious eyes of anesthesiologists. The chest rose, then fell. Quick check for a carotid pulse—just below the jawline, right where they'd seen it back at the morgue—showed no heartbeat at all. They started compressions right there on the floor. This was the kind of place ambulance cops had once avoided and the morticians in their hearses refused to go, the kind of patient who without Freedom House would get no treatment, no transport, no nothing. Still, it can be a hopeless feeling to crunch away on a lifeless chest. Beating for a heart with a million reasons to stop.

But Rayzer and Morant kept going, these children of the Father of CPR, working their patient all the way to Presby, where later he'd stand to walk out, dazed but resurrected, confirmation that miracles can happen among us.

THIS WAS NOVEMBER 1968. Five months before, on July 15, a call had gone out for a woman with seizures on a city bus at the 3900 block of Forbes Avenue. She was transported without incident to Presby, and her routine and largely unremarkable emergency marked the official start of the Freedom House Ambulance Service, the first call for a corps of medics that would, in short order, begin showing the way for a nation in need of change.

But plenty of work remained.

Freedom House had coasted through training on financial fumes. Hallen worked furiously to raise money, and by July his efforts began to bear fruit. He got money from the Ford Foundation, the Richard King Mellon Foundation, and the Kaufmann Foundation. The city kicked in, and so did the US Labor Department and the Office of Economic Opportunity. He raised enough money to last six weeks, then kept on going until there was enough, about $300,000, to operate through the end of the year. Their agreement with the city to provide twenty-four-hour ambulance service in the Hill District and the adjoining neighborhood of Oakland was covered financially but only just barely.

If the medics knew about Freedom House's dire financial situation, they didn't let it affect the quality of care they delivered. In the first year alone, they responded to nearly six thousand calls and were credited with saving more than two hundred of their neighbors from heart attacks, gunshots, stabbings, and overdoses. Their average arrival time was under ten minutes, and in nearly every case they delivered that patient to the hospital alive.

When not on calls, they served as walking billboards for the service, turning out in their pressed white uniforms to show off their equipment to society women from Squirrel Hill or teach local residents how to perform CPR. A second class of paramedic students followed the first, and within the year, nineteen more men would hit the streets.

By the spring of 1969, the new ambulances Safar first conceived of years before started rolling in. Ford Econoline vans like the Mystery Machine. They cost thirteen grand apiece, with a crown of lights and sirens ringing the top and an orange-and-white paint scheme that would be adopted by other services for decades to come. Each had a large emblem on the side door that read, "Freedom House Ambulance."

Safar was a pioneer in the burgeoning field of critical care medicine and, after arriving in Pittsburgh, started what is considered America's first ICU. He envisioned Freedom House as a critical aspect of advanced care and referred to these new ambulances as mobile ICUs or MICUs. They were modified and equipped to exceed national recommendations—admittedly a low bar—and carried wall-mounted suction units, portable oxygen and airway equipment, defibrillators and cardiac monitors, plus all the splinting and bandaging gear you could dream up. As he'd insisted, there was room to spare, with a seat at the head of the stretcher where a single medic could command and control patient care all the way to the hospital.

That same year, Freedom House also added a third precinct, downtown, to its area of control. The dream of a first-class ambulance service was finally coming true. If they were outrunning initial expectations and proving to be far more than a jobs program for young men from a poverty-stricken neighborhood, then the reason was, as Hallen foresaw, that it was not just for but *of* the people it served. A sense of ownership stretched from the mechanics and dispatchers all the way up to leadership. Pride came as much from what they did as from who was doing it.

The base station at Presby was full of big personalities, but the largest of all was night shift supervisor Walt Brown. Walt was impossible to ignore. He was big and loud, sucked all the air out of the room, then breathed his own back into it. You didn't have to figure Walt out; he'd tell you who he was. Player, gambler, ladies' man. He would tell people he'd been a hoodlum, been in jail, been to Nam. A guy with the imposing physical presence to be both charming and menacing all at once. He was a man in perpetual motion, always searching for an angle and forever in the midst of a crisis. Trouble with a new girl or an old girl or both at once. One of them needed a new car or a new air conditioner, a new job—anything—and there was Walt, saddled with the problem and looking for an answer, telling you about it as he went.

There was Curtis Scott, a former bookie and gambler in his midsixties, who joined Freedom House because he didn't have Social Security and wanted something to pass on to his kids. Harvey Gandy was a former cab driver who could pick a car lock in the snap of a finger. Ron Ragin was there, quiet and understated, with the air of an accountant, and so was Pearl Porter, a dispatcher who talked as much off the phone as on. It was an eccentric group, something that felt like family, with everyone coming together for the same vital purpose.

Their immediate and unqualified success meant to the Freedom House board that while ambulance companies were rapidly going out of business, their public/private model worked. To City Hall it meant the police weren't the only ones who could handle the growing number of emergency calls. To Safar it meant simply that lives would be saved. He fired off a letter to the mayor urging him to expand the program. "The time for action has come," he wrote.

In the Hill, Freedom House went beyond the practical or tangible. To their community, the paramedics were souls of a common struggle whose meaning and importance need not be quantified or explained—a candle is more than a flicker when you've been lost in the darkness. "It was the biggest thing," described Lorraine Green, who lived in the Hill. "I don't think I'll ever forget the way they made me feel. They all just walked tall—you could tell they were proud of themselves. A lot of us were."

On calls, kids gathered around them. Awe and excitement. Proof, perhaps, that they too might go any direction they chose. The medics themselves felt it too. Arthur Davis, who admitted back in the beginning to having a funny mind, had become obsessed with the job. After just a year, it was his life, his calling. Dave Thomas turned twenty-one on an ambulance and had already helped deliver five babies. Ushering young lives into this world had turned his own around.

The effects of all that success in the first year were wide-ranging, yet perhaps it all came down to this: for far too long, Black men from the Hill had been spoken of and spoken for but rarely heard themselves. Now they were out front—paramedics—leading a movement whose path was uncertain. With each step, and in every way, they were breaking new ground. Arthur Davis summed up the mood in a way that touched all at once the hope and enormity of the moment.

"It makes me . . . proud," he said. "And for my mother, I'm somebody."

CHAPTER NINETEEN

One good year didn't mean Freedom House was out of the woods. As history showed, plenty of EMS organizations had come and gone.

Even though they were now funded through the first year, from the very beginning Freedom House sat on financial quicksand. They were reliant on donations from foundations (which were one-time infusions) and federal grants (which ran out) and city funds (which fluctuated), as well as the $25 fees they billed patients (which weren't going to keep the lights on). But in 1970, Safar stumbled upon a federal program that just might provide an answer. That answer, though, was one that not everybody would like. Maybe that's why, rather than Freedom House manager Bob Zepfel, Safar approached Zepfel's deputy, Mitchell Brown. It's possible that Safar knew selling the medics on this fix wouldn't be easy, and so he went straight to the man many of the crews turned to for leadership.

"Hey, Brown." Safar called out while speeding down the hall. "We need to talk."

Mitch Brown was—and remains—hard to pin down. Equal parts street medic and politician, at once caustic and cautious with his remarks. He started out on an ambulance but quickly moved beyond it, becoming the suit who never quite felt like one. Mitch Brown grew up in the Hill, watching his neighborhood disintegrate around him, burdened and driven by the knowledge that the outside world expected him to fall apart in the same way. But Mitch was determined to escape the trap that had ensnared so many of his friends and neighbors. He graduated from Fifth Avenue High School in 1965 and enrolled at Wayne State University in Detroit. He seemed poised to slip out unscathed until that summer when tragedy struck. One day in August, shortly before Mitch was going to leave for college, his mother collapsed at home.

Mitch laid his mother on the couch, then rushed to call for help. He was upstairs by her side when two white officers strolled in and declared that his mother, who didn't drink, was drunk. He tried to explain the situation, to convey the urgency, the seconds ticking away, but the cops told him they didn't particularly care what he said, and they definitely didn't plan to carry her down the stairs and out to the wagon. So he scooped his mother into his own arms and carried her outside. He laid her on the canvas stretcher, lingering long enough to notice there were holes worn through the floor of the ambulance. While the cops sat up front waiting, Mitch closed the doors. He never again saw his mother alive. She would eventually be diagnosed with a cerebral hemorrhage (after a forty-five-minute wait in the hospital hallway) and die within the week.

That fall he left for Wayne State but only lasted a year before dropping out to enlist in the military. The Air Force turned him into a medic and shipped him off to Vietnam. He came home in '68 without any plans and took stock of what he had to offer—freshly repatriated veteran, Air Force–trained paramedic, tremendous amount of practical experience in a job that (to his knowledge) had no civilian analog. Plus a year's worth of college credits. It was an odd sort of résumé that didn't point in any obvious direction. He began to settle on the idea of becoming an orderly when he caught wind that Peter Safar was in Pittsburgh. This at least was promising. During his medic training, and later in Vietnam, Mitch had learned CPR and the broader points of emergency medicine and resuscitation through Safar's books. He immediately went to Pitt and sought the doctor out. Freedom House was up and running by that point, and Safar eagerly welcomed this ambitious young man into his office and explained the ambulance program. Mitch was shocked. He'd seen the ambulances racing around the Hill but wasn't certain what they were. Now he knew, and he was interested.

"I'm better than anybody you got," he said.

Safar was no stranger to young and arrogant and appreciated the quality when he saw it. He took Mitch straight to the emergency room and, after seeing just how good he really was, hired him on the spot.

Brown might've been cocky, but he was also serious, ambitious, and buttoned-up. From the very start, he set his sights on something higher than riding in the back of an ambulance and quickly worked his way up from medic to crew chief to director of operations. He took pride in hiring people with backgrounds that'd be deal-breakers elsewhere—dishonorable discharges, criminal backgrounds—and giving them a skill. "We're going to make you into a professional," he'd say on hiring new medics.

Behind the pride and the bluster was something deeper. He spent much of his time running calls on people he'd gone to school with, guys who started out just like him but somewhere along the way had zigged when he zagged and wound up gun-shot or overdosed and now lay on the opposite side of the emergency. His desire to keep climbing came with a need to remember. Whatever doors personal success might open, "you can't forget that you've eaten at Eddie's with roaches running around," he said at the time. "When you forget that, you've got problems."

THAT DAY IN Presby, Mitch heard Safar calling to him from behind.

"Hey, Brown. We need to talk."

Mitch was outspoken and direct, not the kind of guy who'd hold his tongue when faced with something he didn't agree with. And surely Safar knew Mitch would disagree with what he had to say: the organization, this groundbreaking Black organization, needed to hire some white people.

Mitch shook his head, adamant. No. The answer was no. "We don't need any white folks—"

Safar listened, his hands in the pockets of his lab coat, ready to deliver the knockout. "We have to do this in order to get money."

"Oh." Mitch was practical above all else. "In that case . . ."

And so, white people.

Why? Richard Nixon. In the early '70s, America was facing crushing inflation and unemployment, and so Nixon pushed through a raft of legislation to combat the problem. He imposed wage and price controls that were wildly unpopular and drew attention from his other efforts, which included federal funds for companies willing to train and hire the waves of unemployed veterans returning from Vietnam. Safar—and now Mitch, as well—immediately recognized this as a lifeline for cash-strapped organizations like Freedom House. That these new hires had to be racially mixed was a hitch, but ultimately not a fatal one.

So Freedom House promptly hired its first white employee. And he promptly quit.

The guy's name has been lost, but as everyone remembers it, he took one look at his coworkers and his patients and the neighborhood he'd be serving, then quickly and without ceremony bolted for the door. This was a problem.

They needed this money. Which meant they needed a white guy good enough to do the job and who wasn't scared of the neighborhood. Or the patients. Or his own coworkers. They had no idea where to find such a guy but—because serendipity is everywhere in the Freedom House story—they wouldn't have to. As luck would have it, the right guy was already looking for them.

AT THAT VERY moment and not far away, Bill Raynovich was trying to find his way home. Like thousands of other freshly discharged veterans considering their next steps, nothing in Raynovich's upbringing prepared him for military service or for that matter what to do with himself when it was over. He grew up in McKeesport, a suburb of Pittsburgh so small it's basically unknown to anyone not from there. His childhood was sleepy, noteworthy only for being so typically unnoteworthy in its middle-class Americanness. His lone brush with the fantastic happened, coincidentally enough, on an ambulance. It started (as it always does) on a day like any other, when Raynovich returned home from school to find his entire family in the house. There was frantic activity and shouting, everyone panicking. His grandfather, an enormously heavy man, was having a massive heart attack and mixed in with all the usual confusion and hysteria of these situations was anger—it took the ambulance thirty minutes to arrive.

When it finally showed up, everyone had to pitch in to get his grandfather down the steps and out into the ambulance, and in the mad rush to follow it to the hospital they all jumped into their own cars, leaving no one to ride with their patriarch. Bill volunteered. He was just fourteen years old. By now, the song's familiar—you know the words. The attendants tossed his grandfather in the back and hopped up front. Raynovich crawled in next to the stretcher while his grandfather, unattended and moments from death, turned a deep shade of blue. Then came the trip through town, so foreign, so exciting, a space ship ride to eternity. Lights and sirens. Speeding along, running stop lights, weaving through traffic, the world outside a blur. Raynovich was certain beyond all doubt he'd found his future: *I'm going to do this someday.*

After high school, he joined the navy, less out of a sense of patriotism than to avoid getting drafted into the army. He was inducted in February 1967, hoped to land on a battleship or an aircraft carrier, something safe, maybe operating the sonar, but failed the hearing tests and instead wound up a corpsman. He went through basic training and then medical training and after that headed off to California. He was attached to the Fifth Marine Division, Twenty-Eighth Marine Regiment, Second Battalion, Echo Company, Third Platoon. The unit had a storied past—it had fought on Iwo Jima, and its corpsman was believed for a long time to be one of the men raising the American flag atop Mount Suribachi in Joe Rosenthal's famous photo.

All that impressive history was in the past. When Raynovich arrived, the platoon was made up almost entirely of Black men, and several of them, just days before he arrived, were beaten by a group of white marines armed with axe handles. The men of his platoon were so skittish when he got there that they slept with their shovels next to them in bed. For a kid who grew up in a lily-white suburb, it was heavy and disorienting, but Raynovich was nothing if not easygoing, so despite their differences he quickly became just one of the guys. By the summer of '69 he was treating patients—mostly terrified marines attempting to take their own lives—and waiting to get shipped off to Vietnam. Instead, he was somehow spared the deployment and given an honorable discharge the following year. Just like that it was over, and he was back home.

He thought about using the GI Bill to pay for school, but in the meantime decided maybe he'd work on an ambulance. Although he didn't know anything about civilian EMS, he figured surely it had improved since that day he rode alone with his dying grandfather. Turns out, it hadn't. He walked into the offices of a small suburban ambulance company and was told, despite his training—which as a corpsman was something akin to the modern physician's assistant—that he'd first have to take a thirty-hour first aid course. He explained his training and credentials, but nobody understood what he was saying, and anyway, they didn't provide any of the treatment he was qualified to deliver. He left frustrated and bewildered. His mother began searching for an ambulance service that could use someone with her son's advanced skills and came across Cyril Wecht—the Allegheny County coroner and famed forensic pathologist who disputed the Warren Commission's findings in the assassination of John F. Kennedy.

Wecht suggested Raynovich call Safar.

It's hard to guess, as he sat across from Raynovich, what Safar thought of this gangly kid with the scraggly beard and big open smile who'd plopped himself down in his office. Surely Safar was hopeful that they'd found their (white) man and, by extension, their slice of Nixon's new funding initiative. But Safar had already been bitten once by someone who promised he could handle the job, and this time he wanted to be sure. He was casual, affable, but all the while probing into Raynovich's background and personality, looking for glimpses into what made this kid tick and whether he'd be able to hack it. Raynovich knew just enough about Freedom House to pick up on this, and he quickly set Safar at ease, explaining how he'd already served as the token white guy once and had no problem with doing it again.

Safar gave Raynovich his blessing and sent him down to see Zepfel, who was much more skeptical. Zepfel didn't care for a repeat of their past failure and, washing his hands of it, passed Raynovich off on someone else. It went on like this—nobody really sure what to do with him and everyone trying to dodge responsibility—until, finally, Raynovich was given an interview. Sort of. To him it felt more as if they were looking for a reason not to hire him but couldn't find one, and so instead he was handed a uniform and told to come back in the morning.

For his new coworkers, being part of an all-Black organization had special meaning. Few had envisioned that something like it was even possible, and the pride they got from going into Black communities, their own communities, and bringing hope would stand as the crowning achievement of their careers. Freedom House wasn't just a job for them; it was a passion, an organization to which they owed a great debt. They weren't eager to see it change, and when Raynovich walked in, he represented change. Many were skeptical about the white people showing up—what were their motives, where were their loyalties, did they understand just how special this place was? Ultimately, it would come down to trust.

If Raynovich was being sized up, he never felt it. He acted as if he belonged, and to his surprise, it seemed he did. In the dispatch room, on the trucks, nobody batted an eye. If medicine teaches you anything, it's that we all bleed red and die easy, and for the Freedom House crews, only one thing really mattered: When everything went wrong, as it frequently did, and all hell broke loose, could they trust him to hold his own and have their backs? From his first day, on one call after another, Raynovich proved that they could.

And that was that. The ambulances had hit a speed bump, and once again they kept going.

CHAPTER TWENTY

By 1972, Freedom House employed thirty-five crew members and was running seven thousand calls a year. The world began to take note of what was happening in Pittsburgh. The National Research Council liked the training course so much they suggested every EMS service adopt it. Meanwhile Safar, along with Jerry Esposito and Freedom House medical director Don Benson, started the National Registry of Emergency Medical Technicians to help formalize the field and left it in the stewardship of the American Medical Association in Columbus, Ohio. The National Registry continued to grow in scope and influence, and it remains *the* governing body of national EMS standards in America to this day. Find a paramedic in the United States, and you'll find a corresponding National Registry number.

Before long, Freedom House innovations were everywhere. Since Safar's specially designed ambulances first hit the streets in 1969, services nationwide had been swapping their old hearse-style units for these newer, more spacious and intuitive models. The ambulance was just the beginning. Back in the late '50s, Safar had partnered with toy manufacturer Asmund Laerdal to create a CPR mannikin called Resusci Anne, and now he had Laerdal make a new mannikin capable of recording the frequency and efficacy of a trainee's rescue breaths and chest compressions, thereby making training more realistic and effective. Freedom House also reintroduced doctors to ambulance work, both through regular radio communication between crews in the field and physicians in the hospital, and by designating one doctor to provide guidance and education for an ambulance program. Decades later, doctors serving as medical directors would remain a cornerstone of the industry.

Beyond training and transportation, they were also on the cutting edge of the type of gear medics used in the field. Freedom House field-tested early versions of the air cast (for quick and easy splinting of fractures) and the stair chair (an easy-to-carry stretcher that could be folded to negotiate tight corners). In 1967, Miami's Dr. Eugene Nagel introduced something called telemetry that allowed medics to transmit EKGs obtained on their ambulances back to doctors in the hospital. It was very space-age and exciting, and of course Freedom House jumped on it right away.

Every day Safar and the medics were shredding some new convention and turning one or another of medicine's long-held expectations on its head. Take the city's nurses. It wasn't long ago that nurses had barred Freedom House entry into the OB wing and handed them mops in the emergency room, but now it was the nurses who were being sent to *them* for training. The nursing program at Sewickley Hospital recognized that walking into and around a patient's house gave paramedics an unparalleled understanding not only of how that patient lived but also of the factors that led to their current emergency. So nursing students rode along on Freedom House ambulances to get a close-up view of their patients' environment and a few pointers on consoling anxious family members and controlling angry bystanders.

The nursing students (it was the 1970s, so they were women) were almost all young and from the suburbs. They showed up wide-eyed and scared, but quickly warmed to the task—and the medics. Asked for a reaction, one nurse ecstatically described the men who rode alongside her into danger as "fabulous! They are so cool!" You see where this is going. Young students let loose on an adventure. Excitement. Danger. A swaggering paramedic to guide the way. Sometimes they slept together. It was a collision of cultures, but brief, and whatever sparked during the ride-alongs ended when the nurses left the Hill and returned to their quiet suburban lives. Not so for the medics.

As emissaries of this new and remarkable field, their outreach never stopped. They headed west to visit Kansas City, north to New York and Connecticut. When an International Symposium on EMS was planned in Mainz, Germany, Safar asked Mitch Brown to join him. Mitch said no—the Steelers were playing—but eventually buckled under pressure, and the two of them headed off to Mainz. There, at the University of Gutenberg, they were part of a presentation that convinced a panel of experts from around the world "that there is no evidence of reduced mortality and morbidity with advanced life-support rendered by physicians riding ambulances versus well-trained [paramedics.]" Translation: when all hell broke loose and a patient's life was on the line, anything a doctor could do, a medic could do (as well, if not) better.

THIS PRONOUNCEMENT WASN'T merely academic. At the time, Pittsburgh was in the midst of a ballooning heroin epidemic and a corresponding surge in overdoses. But looking around, people noticed heroin-related deaths were climbing in white neighborhoods even as they were dropping in Black ones. The reason was simple. Safar had taken a drug then used only to reverse anesthesia in operating rooms—Narcan—and issued it to his medics. In a scene whose echoes continue to this day, Freedom House medics crouched on the floor of shooting galleries and back alleys across their territory injecting Narcan, which rapidly and dramatically got their lifeless patients breathing again.

Overdoses were just the tip. Over a two-month period in 1972, doctors surveyed more than fourteen hundred patients Freedom House had delivered to area hospitals. In critical patients, Freedom House medics provided appropriate care 89 percent of the time. Compare that to the police, who in the same study were found to have delivered *the wrong care* 62 percent of the time. The numbers were even worse among volunteer ambulance services that did the wrong thing an astounding *87 percent of the time.*

Naturally, this started conversations about setting stricter training standards. Police and fire departments, funeral homes, volunteer services, all viciously fought off any attempts to increase training. They almost always claimed such standards would be too costly, but here again Freedom House proved them wrong. A Freedom House crew, which was paid less than their counterparts in the police, had gotten more than three hundred hours of training (compared to the twenty-five to eighty everyone else got) and arrived on-scene with a defibrillator, cardiac monitor, telemetry, a drug box, and suction, bandaging, and splinting equipment. All on a shoestring budget. And Safar's state-of-the-art ambulance? It cost much less than the city's police wagons.

Freedom House was growing and adapting—chameleon and trendsetter and source of pride all wrapped up in one—and it was on their impressive doors, early in the summer of 1972, that John Moon came knocking for a second time.

BOOK THREE

CHAPTER TWENTY-ONE

On his very first shift at Freedom House, John was dispatched to a person down, possibly not breathing. The second they got in the ambulance, his partner asked if he knew CPR, which John took to mean they were about to perform it, and so, without a word, he scrambled into the back and opened the packaging on every piece of equipment they'd need for a cardiac arrest—plus stuff they wouldn't. When they pulled up on-scene, the patient was standing there talking, a smile on his face, nothing wrong with him at all. This happens in EMS: people call for every reason, sometimes no reason. That his patient was standing and not dying was a good thing for everyone except John. All the equipment he'd opened now had to be brought back to the hospital for sterilization. Freedom House had only a couple crews, and rather than getting back in service, John had to replace all the equipment on his truck. On his first day, before he'd run a single real call, he was dragged into his supervisor's office. It wasn't the impression he'd hoped to make.

Months back, when he first barged into Harold Holland's office, only to be sent away frustrated and embarrassed, John went right out and enrolled in a newly established course over at Community College of Allegheny County, which had formed a loose partnership with Freedom House. He was one of only several students, a few of whom dropped out. It was a slog. He juggled class hours with shifts at Montefiore, plus having a family and a life (kinda). But he was determined to succeed, and he did. Then he went back to Presby and took the test.

This time he sat across from Mitch Brown, who shook his hand and welcomed him aboard. John was officially a Freedom House medic. He was issued uniforms and given a shift and a start date. "You can work nights—come in tomorrow."

When he got home, he snuck off into the bedroom he and Betty shared. There, with nobody watching—it was the orphanage all over again, dancing to Jackie Wilson on the radio in secret—he slipped the uniform on and stood in front of the mirror. It was an intense moment. Pride doesn't cover it. Whatever affirmation or sense of achievement he'd gotten from all those alpaca sweaters, the gold jackets, it was nothing like this. Through all the bed pans, the steel mill, April '68, the counselors, and the long, quiet ride to Pittsburgh, way back to when he was in the orphanage, he swore that someday he'd be something, and now at last he was.

He arrived for his first shift terrified. As an orderly, he'd been regarded with an indifferent anonymity occasionally broken by suspicion. He couldn't do a thing unless he was told, but now he was expected to know what needed to be done and then just do it. He was still working his way through a shyness that had plagued him since Atlanta, and here he was supposed to speak up and take charge. And then there was the intimidation factor of the other guys working there, most of them young and overconfident, everybody talking or laughing all at once, nobody giving much thought to the new guy.

John had blown that first call, so he desperately wanted to get one under his belt, a good one—death and mayhem, blood everywhere—just to get it out of the way, so everyone would know he could handle it.

It was early evening a few days later when that call came in.

To the west, the sky held a flash of sun, but everywhere else it was darkening to purple. Pearl Porter hung up the dispatch phone, her welcoming face at odds with the details she was trying to deliver. Fire at the Bedford Dwellings, just one apartment but fully engulfed. An elderly woman trapped inside. The words hit like a tingle at the base of

John's spine and sent him running out the door. Even with everything he had learned about burns, how to quantify and treat them, flashing through his head, he didn't feel ready. Not for a real burn, if that's what this was. A dump of adrenaline blazed a jangled trail for the nerves, but no endorphins followed to send his mind down that calming path. There was only fear. The two-way radio chattered in his ear and filled the ambulance with anxious noise that only made it worse. The fire department requested another engine be sent. Then another. The ambulance crested a hill and came barreling down the other side, brake pads worn to nothing, so even with his partner practically standing on the pedal—brakes screaming all the way—John wasn't sure they'd stop before crashing through an intersection or, worse, hurtling off the edge into the water.

John was only a few days on the job and scared as hell, afraid he'd make a mistake, and too alone to tell anyone about it. His partner, driving, not looking, not talking, was opaque, a face without a name. They didn't talk, really. Certainly John didn't talk, just stayed quiet most of the time and spoke when spoken to, kept whatever he was feeling (terror, mostly) to himself. There was no one he could turn to and say, "I'm not ready for this." It was too late for that anyhow.

They rounded a corner, and the Bedford Dwellings came into view. It was the city's first housing project, labeled a great experiment when it opened in 1940 on eighteen acres of the Hill District overlooking the Allegheny River. Before that it was Greenlee Field—home of the Crawfords—and before that a cemetery. Its four hundred twenty apartments were once the most sought-after public housing in the city. Now mothers chased drug dealers from the halls with brooms. The buildings faced one another with courtyards in between, and as John and his partner wove their way around the collection of ladder trucks and engines that had responded to the multi-alarm fire, they watched the scene with growing disorientation.

Hoses snaked in every direction. Firefighters were everywhere. Chiefs and captains, their underlings. Operating the trucks, opening hydrants, raising a ladder so they could shoot water from above. Firefighters with hand lines running toward the building, and then, from inside, guys rushing back out. The ones coming out, though, weren't holding hoses. They had a person.

John wasn't really there in that moment; he'd slipped from participant to spectator. As if the whole thing was happening somewhere else and he wasn't part of it. But these firefighters kept coming toward him, and as they got closer, their blurry cargo took the form of a woman. Elderly. Burned horribly and not moving. John wondered what they would do for her, what they even *could* do, when his partner yanked open the back doors of the ambulance, and suddenly the firefighters were inside and the woman was on their stretcher. Finally, John snapped out of it—or maybe into it. This patient was his. What happened to her now was up to him. And just like that, his day went from bad to worse.

"Burns are third-degree." He said it aloud but to himself, really. His partner, less new than John but still new, was already backing away. "Eighty-five percent of her body. This isn't good."

Burns—whether from water or the stove—are classified into three categories and rated by severity. For this woman, trapped in her apartment as the flames and smoke crept toward her, they would've come on in stages.

First-degree burns are the most superficial: mild (think of a sunburn) and often caused by radiant heat. With flames licking at the walls, the air inside the apartment would've gotten hotter and hotter until her skin, drained of moisture, began to redden and grow tender. The next stage, second-degree, would've come as the flames drew closer and occasionally lashed out. A second-degree burn penetrates the outer layer of the skin, called the epidermis, to reach the fat below. The skin swells and begins to blister. Maybe it bursts. Whatever panic this might cause is only heightened by the super-heated air, which by now would be searing her lungs with each gasping breath. At this point her condition was still reversible.

But the flames kept coming.

The last stage, the one now staring John in the face, is third-degree. A full-thickness burn. The flesh chars white, and everything beneath—bones, tendons, vessels—they're all burned. Nerve endings, too—a small miracle because at least the pain of being scorched alive was over. By this point John's patient would've been blanketed in flames that sucked up all the oxygen and left nothing but carbon monoxide, which would surely have knocked her out. Whether someone can be saved at this point depends, in part, on just how much of their body surface has been burned. The limbs and torso, the head, they're all assigned a percentage of the total. The head accounts for 9 percent, and it's 18 for the legs. The torso is 36. That John's patient had burns over 85 percent of her body suggests all areas were partially hit and others had burned entirely.

He looked up. The firefighters were gone. It was just the two Freedom House paramedics and their patient. Her clothes burned off, jewelry still on. John reached down and touched the necklace on her chest. It was hot.

"We gotta get this off." He looked up; he looked down, thinking of how her body would eventually swell. "There's gonna be edema, and this is gonna be difficult to remove when we get to the hospital, and it could turn into a tourniquet and . . ."

And now John was beginning to spin out, losing himself somewhere near the edge of panic. Time slowed; a thousand things raced through his mind. None of them helpful. He got to work, starting with the rings, but they wouldn't budge so he went for the bracelets, but the woman's skin—with that full-thickness burn—started coming off in his bare hands.

"Oh." He shook his head, hands full of hot jewelry and loose flesh. "Let's—let's just get out of here. Go, just go."

He wasn't thinking right. Neither was his partner. They were shaken and rushed and no longer bordering on panic but fully there. Rather than going to Mercy Hospital, the burn center, they went instead to Presby. As soon as they walked in, the doctors, furious—"Why did you bring her here?!"—started the process of transferring her to Mercy. Another Freedom House ambulance had to be sent to fix their mess, which everyone could see. There was no way to hide it. None of this changed the patient's outcome. There wasn't much John could've done had he kept it together; her prognosis was terrible, and even the experienced medics couldn't have done much better. Still, he hadn't done right by this patient. He was now a fully trained Freedom House paramedic, with all the responsibility and pride that badge entailed, and he hadn't done his job. As soon as he cleared the hospital, John was called in to see his supervisor. Bad news piled on bad news.

Will Holland, the brother of the guy who'd originally told John he wasn't qualified for the job, was now his boss. Holland was strict and intimidating, and John hadn't exactly proven himself. First it was the guy who wasn't unconscious, and now this. John stood there alongside his partner getting chewed out by Will Holland. Pick an insult or a cuss word, any spit-inflected way to vent your rage, and that's what Holland was hurling at them now. Their first and foremost sin was panicking, which would've been bad enough on its own, but they went and followed it up by going to the wrong hospital and making Freedom House look bad.

John didn't even know Mercy was a burn center. But this was life and death: it didn't really matter what you had or hadn't been told. As Holland railed on, John didn't feel defeat or even the embarrassment he'd felt after opening all that sterilized equipment. What he felt was disappointment. Holland's disappointment in him. John stood there and took the ass-chewing, but when it was over he didn't dwell on it long. Couldn't. He had to make it up and prove himself before it was too late. All those years he spent looking for a way to make his mark, and now that he got it, everything was slipping through his fingers.

It was then, as everything seemed to be coming undone, that he was partnered with George McCary. And from there, it all began to change.

George McCary joined Freedom House in 1968, with the second class of trainees and perfectly fit the profile of a wild young man who'd found himself in this unlikeliest of places. He wasn't looking for a job when he joined. He didn't even want a job, definitely didn't want to go back to school. All he wanted was to hang out and meet girls, but he'd already been kicked out of his girlfriend's place and was now on the verge of getting kicked out of his grandmother's house too. Girls came around too much and made themselves at home. His grandmother had enough.

"You got to go," she told him.

"Where am I supposed to go?"

"It don't matter. You got to go. Either get a job or go to school."

One of George's cousins worked at Freedom House and told him how the recruiters plucked people off the street with a promise to turn their lives around with a job that would use their minds instead of their backs. This caught his attention. Guys like him mostly disappeared into the steel mills for thirty years of toil. George saw himself as a hustler, and this ambulance thing, from the pitch right on down to the job itself, sounded like a hustle. He signed on. His grandmother was skeptical. She figured he'd wash out before the training was done but agreed to let him stay in her house as long as he actually went to class. George was undisciplined and didn't like structure, but he took the deal.

"I'm not doing this for me," he told her. "I'm doing it to show you I can."

In the end he showed everybody. George fell in love with it on the first day and never looked back. He was only just out of training the first time he slipped a man into a body bag. He'd never been so close to a corpse, had never done something so important. It felt immediate and vital. He loved that he understood the human body, that it was his job to fix it when something went wrong. He hated the smells and the mess—between all the sweat and blood he went through two uniforms a night—but he liked that there was always the chance of touching a moment that felt close to grace. A new life, an ending life, a second chance at life. One night he saved a man with CPR and later, at the hospital, stood there just watching him talk to the doctors. George had done that with his own hands. He struggled to explain the emotion (a rare moment of quiet) but knew he'd found his way into something deep.

Unlike some of the other guys who arrived in '68, George didn't get promoted. He still enjoyed the life he had outside work, and even on the ambulance he was never serious. By his own estimation, he wasn't management material, and that was fine with him. But he had a sort of genius for the chaos of the job, an easygoing way even under pressure. Like water. George flowed with the moment. Maybe that's why, after he'd been with Freedom House a few years, he was partnered with John, who never flowed.

They were beyond opposites. John so serious he described himself as "starchy" as if it were a compliment. He was thin and stiff as a board, and now here came George, a thick guy with a rolling gait and that easy smile. He joked all the time and willingly admitted that even his grandmother didn't believe he'd make it at Freedom House. "But I came out smelling like a rose," George would say with a laugh. "When you're the chosen one like me, opportunity comes." He loved people, loved talking. He was always talking. One thing people would remember about George was how he never took anything seriously, no matter how serious it was.

From the moment they started working together, the McCary magic was on display.

"Hey man! How's it going?"

George walked right up and slapped hands with their patient—middle-aged man in the road, altered mental status. They found him not far from Mercy Hospital. It went like this on calls: John focused and serious, George off talking to whomever he knew on the scene. And he knew everybody, like he was the mayor. If he recognized a bystander, he'd wander off and talk to them. This time he knew the patient. The guy was a drunk, George said. This corner was his spot. He started goofing around with the guy, acting as if he were drunk too. John, fresh off a reprimand and determined to prove himself to Holland, set down their jump bag and started his physical exam. George laughed as John took the guy's pulse and blood pressure. He checked his sugar and was assessing him for evidence of head trauma when he noticed George had gotten quiet. John glanced over his shoulder to see George standing there in his approximation of a *very serious look*, his face straight, voice somber. George nodded. Maybe John was right. Maybe it was head trauma, a brain bleed. Something deadly.

Then his face broke into a huge smile. *Or* maybe the guy was drunk. George burst out laughing, then wheeled around to the patient, who was laughing now too. John shook his head. It was clear, even to him, the guy was just drunk. You could smell him across the street. Light a match, and they'd all be gone. John allowed a small laugh at his own self-seriousness to slip out.

"There you go." George slapped his arm. "Just gotta lighten up a little."

John did lighten up. A little. George's laughing and joking, his inability to take anything seriously at all, forced John to relax, and once he relaxed, he was finally able to do the work. He got used to the ambulance, the equipment, the crowds. He learned to tell the critical from the dramatic and how to deliver care in the street. George changed, too. On-scene he was still the jester and ringleader, the soother of frayed nerves, but he came to trust John's instinct and sometimes, though not always, kept his focus. He got rowdy bystanders to calm down and frantic family members to carry equipment. On the scene of an overdose, he'd track down the dealer (he knew *everyone*) to figure out what the guy had taken and assure everyone that his partner, John—*that's the doctor, there*—would take care of the problem.

There were no limits to his charm. And so there were light moments, but there was also redemption. Not long after they started working together, they were dispatched to a critical patient at the Bedford Dwellings, the same eighteen acres of brick apartments overlooking the Allegheny where John fumbled the burn patient. This time everything went the way it was supposed to.

Ease bred success, and with each win John grew more confident. The shell he'd retreated into years before cracked wide open, and finally he could breathe. He started talking in the station and made friends and even managed to resurrect his relationship with Holland. He wasn't scared anymore; he didn't panic. The job was coming to him now. It still wasn't easy, but it felt natural. Less like what he was paid to do and more like what he was born to do. He finally understood the job that just a year before, when he first walked into Holland's office had been such a mystery. He ran hundreds of calls his first year, affected dozens of lives, and right there, on the very streets where he'd once felt so alone and inconsequential, he found his place. John Moon was home.

But no home is perfect.

CHAPTER TWENTY-TWO

In the early hours of January 12, 1972, on a street corner in the Homewood section of Pittsburgh, a young man named Michael Blackman was shot and killed. What Blackman was doing out there in the dark is uncertain, but some facts are clear. It was after four in the morning, just thirty degrees, and he was by himself as a passing car slowed in the street. Behind the wheel was a twenty-nine-year-old Brooklyn man named George Harrington whom Blackman allegedly owed $1,100 for drugs. When Harrington saw him, he stopped the car and got out. From there things got out of hand quickly.

Neighbors said they heard fighting. Harrington later said that Blackman slapped him, that he opened his jacket and reached for a knife, and at that point, fearing for his life, Harrington pulled out his gun. The police never found a knife. What they found was Blackman's "bullet-ridden" body on the sidewalk, shot through the chest and hands. Michael Blackman was twenty-four when he was killed, a husband and father of two. He was also one of the young men pulled off the streets of the Hill District and enrolled in the original paramedic class back in 1967. He joined Freedom House to escape a troubled past only for it to catch up with him on the corner of Tyson and Baxter streets.

His murderer was arrested almost by accident—swept up a few days later in a drug sting in East Liberty that netted $50,000 worth of heroin and five suspects. As the cops rushed in, Harrington threw a .38-caliber pistol to the ground, one of four guns picked up in the bust, that ballistics experts later identified as the weapon used to kill Blackman. It was pretty much a straight line from there. A confession, then conviction, then sentencing—each tugged along by the others as if tied together on a short string. At Freedom House, the reaction to the conviction and sentencing of Blackman's killer was subdued. His murder wasn't the first. Two years earlier, Carl Staten—another graduate of the first class—had been killed by his wife in a domestic dispute. Nobody talked much about Blackman's death, and it struck John as strange. Even George McCary, who had something to say about everything, in this case had almost nothing to say at all. The medics seemed almost relieved to move on.

Truth is, despite their success, it had not been an easy run for Freedom House. Maybe John was too new and excited, so proud just to be there, that he hadn't noticed the cracks, but for everyone who'd been there from the beginning, the sting of Blackman's murder was just one in a series of challenges dogging them almost from the very beginning. Freedom House had now been on the streets for four years, a span that carried the country not only into a new decade but into a different era altogether.

America had changed since 1968. Or hadn't, depending on how you saw it. Surely something had faded. The high-minded euphoria of the '60s, the feeling that enough Baby Boomers—the largest generation the country had ever seen—saw things for how they were and wanted to make them better and that together all those people could not be stopped: those days now seemed almost like a dream. "We had all the momentum; we were riding the crest of a high and beautiful wave," was how Hunter S. Thompson described it after all that hope had bled out into the '70s. "So now, less than five years later . . . with the right kind of eyes you can almost see the high-water mark—that place where the wave finally broke and rolled back."

There wasn't a single moon that pushed back the tide, but Richard Nixon's 1968 presidential election drew its share of water. His campaign seemed like a national turning away from Johnson's Great Society and the War on Poverty and toward an appeal to what he would call the "silent majority," those working- and middle-class white voters tired of the turbulence, of the riots and antiwar protests, the counterculture, the civil rights movement, a government of liberals that meddled too much in their lives. His was a conservative brand of populism, professing to be against both big government and big business, but succeeding mainly in being Us versus Them.

Claiming to speak for the "forgotten Americans, the non-shouters, the non-demonstrators," people who felt under siege during the "long, dark night" of the '60s, Nixon said, "Enough is enough," and America—faced with a weakening economy, a wider war in Vietnam, oil embargoes, the Manson murders (shortly), and a general sense that somehow the country had lost its way—agreed with him. He won the popular vote by the narrowest of margins. His election meant an end to the presidential commissions and the antipoverty programs and the start of official resistance from Washington to desegregation and busing initiatives. Soldiers who'd left an America full of drugs and free love and hippies and music returned just a year later—confused and a little horrified—to find it awash in polyester and sideburns.

As usual, Pittsburgh was right there, if not leading the train then certainly riding it. In 1969, the city elected a populist of its own, an anti-establishment mayor whose ideas about how things should be done would put Freedom House squarely in City Hall's crosshairs.

WITH BOOS AND jeers from a thousand-odd protestors raining down, Peter Flaherty had to raise his voice to keep from being drowned out. It was January 5, 1970, a cold Pittsburgh day, and Flaherty, speaking from the steps of City Hall, had just been sworn in as mayor. In a

Kennedy-esque gesture, he wore no coat as he spoke about civil rights, about law and order, about change and a new day for the city, a philosophy reflected in his swearing in, which, for the first time since 1934, was open to the public and held in the rotunda rather than in council chambers. Flaherty was forty-four, tall, handsome, and broad-shouldered. Beside him stood his wife, Nancy, a former beauty queen. He was a self-styled maverick, and many Pittsburghers saw him as a breath of fresh air who promised a housecleaning upon arrival. The protesters were there because he'd lived up to that promise, firing the long-serving police superintendent before he was even in office, a move that angered the city's cops and whose ghost would at least partially explain—to early supporters who'd later become opponents—some of his behavior in years to come. But that January day, Flaherty represented a clean break from the past.

Born on June 24, 1924, Pete Flaherty was fairly typical for white Pittsburgh—Irish, child of immigrants, raised on the North Side, where his family ran a grocery store. He was stationed in Guam during World War II, a navigator on B-29s who flew missions over Japan. After V-J Day he returned home, went to law school, and worked as an assistant district attorney. It was there that he caught the eye of Mayor Joseph Barr, who personally selected him for a vacant seat on the city council. It was a decision the mayor most likely later regretted. When Barr decided not to seek a third term, Flaherty took on the party's chosen candidate in the Democratic primary, bucking the political machine that had anointed every mayor since the Great Depression.

Running under the slogan "Nobody's Boy," Flaherty won the primary in a landslide. The party tried to make amends and mailed him thousands of campaign stickers for the general election. The gesture failed—he and Nancy were photographed throwing the stickers in the trash. That November he won the general election, ushering in what one observer called a whole new style of politics. He was a populist Democrat but a fiscal conservative, an opponent of big business, labor unions, and interest groups. He was against public-private partnerships, believing instead that all public programs and infrastructure projects should be controlled by the government itself—cheaply when possible, shut down when not.

Right out of the gate he got rid of about two thousand city employees—including someone whose job it was to clean the spittoons in City Hall—launched his opposition to a major transit project, and, of course, fired the police superintendent. Freedom House was next.

CHAPTER TWENTY-THREE

Just days after his inauguration, Flaherty's public safety director, James Cortese, announced the city would slash the amount of money paid to the ambulance service in half. Rather than a hundred grand per year, Freedom House would now get just fifty. Cortese was quick to point out this wasn't done because of some deficiency on Freedom House's part; in fact he said, "The service is excellent," and hoped "to talk Freedom House Enterprises into continuing coverage" at the current level. They'd just have to do it with half the money. If they refused, then the cops would take over, meaning that medics whose training and experience made them perhaps the most highly skilled ambulance units in the country would be replaced by police officers with a week's worth of training.

To everyone involved with Freedom House, this was unthinkable. For Safar, who'd finally carved out a toehold in the critical world of street medicine, ceding it to the cops was out of the question, and as for the medics, there was no way in hell they were retreating. They'd given too much, and it was too important—to them and to the community. The service was theirs, and they wouldn't return to the days when the cops refused to carry Mitch Brown's mother to the ambulance. Even stripped of emotion, the very idea boggled the mind. In the past year alone, Freedom House responded to seventy-seven strokes, more than a hundred twenty women in labor, and nearly two hundred seizure patients. They'd recently been sent to a man in cardiac arrest and, using their defibrillator, shocked him back to life. When that man walked out of the hospital three weeks later, it was believed by some to be the first time an ambulance crew had pulled off such a feat.

And yet the incoming mayor saw them simply as a jobs program, a line item on the city budget to be finessed or removed at will. So Safar and Hallen and their people got to work, raising more money from private sources to keep the lights on. But the mayor remained so determined in his opposition that two years later, when John came on, the fight had reached a boiling point.

HERE THINGS START to get ever more maddening because the city—fronted by the mayor and soon to be joined in this fight by a county commissioner—seemed desperate to get rid of a service that was setting a national curve in medicine. Asked to explain their opposition, they would make every possible excuse, each more specious than the last. Yet the excuses kept coming. It was unnecessary; it was unproven; it was uneconomical; it was un-American (yes, really). They seemed to be saying that government had no business saving the lives of the people it was elected and paid to serve. Maddening.

In 1972, Safar began rattling the mayor's cage. By this point Safar was not only spearheading an effort to bring advanced ambulance care to all of Pittsburgh but had been named head of the governor's Emergency Medical Services Commission, a perch from which he was also demanding statewide action. That his service hadn't been expanded to cover his entire home city drew side-eyed glances. Flaherty was compelled to respond and shrugged off his indifference to Freedom House by saying, "We already have very good ambulance service being performed by the police department." This statement wasn't merely limp; it was demonstrably false.

This *good* service consisted of sixteen police wagons operated by a hundred twenty cops whose ten hours of training didn't include CPR. The ambulances they drove weren't dedicated ambulances but doubled as police vehicles and were prohibitively expensive to replace and so weren't replaced—think back to the holes in the floor of the police wagon that carried Mitch Brown's dying mother. Aside from being old, they didn't meet the minimum design and equipment standards set all the way back in 1968. It was clear to anyone with eyes that what the cops provided wasn't "good."

Safar was backed up here by the ever-present coroner Cyril Wecht, who said, "I get about thirty to fifty cases a year on my autopsy table where I feel good pre-hospital emergency care in ambulances could have saved these people." Many of them, Wecht said, had been transported by the police. These included presumed heart attacks that were actually chokings and presumed drunks that were actually heart attacks. "If they're well-dressed, they're thought to have a heart attack," he said. "If they're unshaven, they're thought to be drunk."

Flaherty might've been satisfied with the police units, but the city's medical experts found them to be "amateurly run" and staffed by attendants with "no training in emergency life-saving methods." They were also unreliable. Don Benson, an anesthesiologist who'd been Freedom House's first medical director, came forward with a story of his own. One afternoon, Benson said, a forty-year-old teacher began having chest pain. As the day wore on, his pain grew more insistent, eventually becoming a heavy pressure under his breastbone. By evening he was sweating heavily, and his wife called the family doctor, who urged her to get him immediately to the hospital. "I'll meet you there," he said. She called the fire department, but they refused to take him to the hospital of their choice. She called the police and got the same answer. Finally, she called a funeral home. The hearse (unequipped) took so long in arriving that her husband was unconscious when the morticians (untrained) walked through the door and dead when he reached the hospital.

He wasn't alone. Safar believed that negligent ambulance care led, countywide, to anywhere from twelve hundred to two thousand preventable deaths a year. He fired off a passionate, uncharacteristically emotional letter to Flaherty. Speaking for the city's dead, he asked the mayor to put himself in their shoes. Imagine, he said, being "severely injured in a traffic accident, picked up like a sack of potatoes, dumped on a canvas stretcher . . . choking to death on your tongue, blood or vomit." The cops likely wouldn't ride in the back with him, but if they did, could he imagine, Safar asked, staring helplessly into the eyes of a man with neither the training nor the equipment to do anything as he drowned in his own vomit? As for whether or not the city's ambulance service was "good," Safar said Flaherty didn't seem to understand the difference between first aid and emergency medicine.

Safar's letter was signed by nearly two dozen medical professionals comprising a citizens' committee on emergency care. He asked for an immediate meeting with Flaherty, or else he'd be forced to make the letter public.

The meeting never happened, and so Safar published the letter. His combative tone drew Allegheny County Commissioner William Hunt into the fight. At fifty-eight, Hunt was a retired surgeon, former coroner, and World War II veteran. He was a musician, a squash player and wine maker, a renaissance man so full of energy his first wife called him "the whirlybird." But he was also known as "an obstructionist," "combative," "never a man to hesitate in standing alone." "If something was new," one colleague noted, "it was suspect." To Hunt, Safar's brand-new paramedics were definitely suspect.

Elected to a body that wielded its power over the entirety of Allegheny County, Hunt arrived at Flaherty's side with significant firepower. And he joined the fight with guns blazing, though at times he seemed confused as to what exactly he was fighting for. When Safar pointed out that deficiencies in the police ambulance system led to Governor Lawrence's death, Hunt accused him of "defaming and insulting" the police. When Safar asked for proof that "the police have passed even the most basic competence test," Hunt shot back that cops were supposed to be doing police work and not driving ambulances. This left everyone scratching their heads. That the police should stick to police work and get out of the ambulance business—which Safar contended they were presently doing to the tune of at least twelve hundred preventable deaths a year—was exactly why he was "defaming and insulting" them in the first place. This, clearly, was not a battle of wits.

If Flaherty and Hunt believed Pittsburgh's police ambulance service to be adequate, they hedged their bet by arguing it was certainly no worse here than anywhere else. Referring to EMS as a "very difficult and controversial medical problem," Hunt suggested that the jury was still very much out on whether street medicine was really a thing. "There are differences of opinion by equally competent medical authorities," he said, "as to the extent of sophisticated medical procedures that can be carried out in an ambulance weaving through busy city streets at fifty to sixty miles an hour." Flaherty called street medicine "a very difficult, complex question."

This, again, was wrong.

Legitimate efforts had been made to improve every facet of EMS—from training to gear to ambulances to public awareness—in at least twenty-four states. Seattle, Atlanta, San Antonio, Detroit, and Houston had all raised their standards. Miami started a paramedic program in 1968, not long after Freedom House. Los Angeles started its own the following year. San Francisco staffed its ambulances with former military medics. Not only were other cities fielding sophisticated ambulance crews similar to Freedom House, but in some areas, Safar's ideas had served as an example. Jacksonville's public safety director was part of both the National Research Council and the National Academy of Sciences—organizations that recommended cities adopt or at least borrow from Freedom House's training program—while Columbus was home to the National Registry of EMTs, which Safar helped to establish.

Since launching their own paramedic programs, Columbus and Jacksonville, each roughly the same size as Pittsburgh, had seen their accident fatality rates drop by 24 and 28 percent respectively. And it was in Columbus that an EMS call provided a stark counterpoint to Benson's cautionary tale. The call involved a fifty-year-old woman named Marie George who had a heart attack at home and slipped into cardiac arrest. Whereas the man in Benson's story died thanks to poor ambulance care, Marie, who later said, "I was clinically dead three times," repeatedly saw the light but never reached it—each time the paramedics dragged her back.

So it wasn't that other cities weren't doing it. Nor was an advanced paramedic corps the sort of luxury only larger towns could pull off. Though it only covered just a small portion of Pittsburgh, the Freedom House training program rivaled or topped that of much bigger cities. San Francisco's repatriated military medics were trained to deal only with cardiac emergencies. Miami's medics had about eighty hours of training, while the paramedics in LA—soon to be lionized in *Emergency!*, a TV show that would inspire a generation of first responders—had a hundred eighty. Each of these cities, all larger than Pittsburgh by a mile, had medics operating with either less training or a narrower scope than Freedom House.

Given that street medicine was being practiced across the country at ever-increasing levels of competence with real and tangible results, that governing bodies at the local, state, and federal level had lifted the bar of acceptable ambulance care from something approaching murderous and then kept on lifting it—to the point that a woman would be snatched from death not once or twice but *three times*—you begin to get the feeling, as one observer noted, that what Hunt referred to as a difference of opinion by "equally competent medical authorities" was in reality only a debate between himself (with Flaherty in tow) and the rest of the American Medical Association.

What do you do in the face of such overwhelmingly rational arguments? Become overwhelmingly irrational in your own. Unable to deny that EMS was in fact thriving all over the country, Flaherty and Hunt adopted perhaps their strangest argument yet—that, legally speaking, both the county and the city were prohibited from running an ambulance service. "The county is not going to get into the ambulance business because we legally can't," Hunt said. "We cannot provide direct [medical] services." Flaherty agreed, saying that "legal concerns" prevented the city from operating ambulances. The problem was that both the county *and* the city were already providing direct medical services, the county through its funding of programs at the Hill House, a local nonprofit, and also at Kane Hospital—procedures that included X-rays and tuberculosis tests and immunizations, even treatment for sexually transmitted diseases—while the city had obviously been administering one ambulance service through the police for twenty years and still another through Freedom House since 1968. Pressed at a city council meeting to explain the discrepancy, Flaherty could only smile.

Maddening.

By 1972, as the mayor dragged his feet, more than $30 million in federal highway money had been spent upgrading ambulance systems around the country. But rather than collect, Pittsburgh allowed $2 million in federal funding to slip away simply because the city never bothered to apply for it. City Councilman Robert Rade Stone urged Flaherty to do something, stating publicly that Pittsburgh was eligible for another million in federal funds and that to get it all Flaherty had to do was apply. There was also private money to be had. The Robert Wood Johnson Foundation, named for the health care titan who founded Johnson & Johnson with his brothers, was in the process of giving away $15 million and had already given financial support to EMS in San Francisco, Philadelphia, Indianapolis, Minneapolis, Cleveland, Atlanta, and Seattle. "I want to make sure the Mayor doesn't pass up this money as he previously did," Stone said.

But Flaherty did pass it up. His reasoning was that most of these grants required the city to chip in money of its own. This he simply wouldn't do. He felt Freedom House should be self-sustaining, a demand made of no other branch of public safety. Without asking for a dime in return, the city spent $19 million a year on the police department and $12 million a year on the fire department. In fact, they spent twice as much money every year on dog catching, about a hundred grand, as they were now spending on Freedom House. *Dog catching.*

What little money they did spend, the city made hard to get. Freedom House board member Paul Williams had to repeatedly harangue the mayor's office about late payment of the $50,000, which the service desperately needed to make weekly payroll but didn't arrive that year until November. Between late payments and the measly $25 fee charged for each transport—often hard to collect in the Hill—the idea of self-sustainability seemed more myth than reality. In fact, the only way to pull it off would've been to expand the service, which would've required not only more money but also City Hall's approval. Citizens' groups in North Side and Hazelwood had already requested Freedom House take over ambulance work, and, of course, expansion into wealthier neighborhoods would've increased the number of calls they ran as well as the chances of getting paid for them. Not to mention the potential for lives saved.

Taking their case to the press, Mitch Brown was quick to point out Pittsburgh's racial disparity in care, though in this instance it was the city's white residents who were suffering. "It doesn't make sense for people to die . . . because of untrained, poorly equipped ambulance attendants, when we could be expanded . . . to serve the entire community," he said. "Right now people in the Hill [get] better emergency care . . . than persons in, say, Squirrel Hill." To change that, meaning to save white lives, Freedom House would need to be expanded. "The need is there, the demand is there, and the supply is there."

By suggesting Freedom House be allowed to move into wealthier neighborhoods, Mitch inadvertently dragged the funeral homes and private ambulance companies into the fight. To those groups, this was a cash cow, not a mission. They argued that government-run services inhibit free enterprise and lobbied against making EMS a public service similar to the police and fire departments. Free emergency medical treatment was socialized medicine, they insisted, and would brainwash people into voting for such dangerous concepts as universal health care. Richard Dixon, head of a company called Tri-Rivers Ambulance, said government funding gave Freedom House an unfair advantage that pushed for-profit services out of business. This, he argued, was "unconstitutional."

Dixon recalled the good old days, "five or six years ago," when Freedom House had "one ambulance [serving] the Hill District because private companies and the police wouldn't go there. Now there are five or six ambulances operating all over the district." The implication was clear: it was fine for Freedom House to cover an area nobody else wanted to cover and help people no one else wanted to help. But the moment they set their sights on wealthier clientele, well, that was unacceptable and possibly even un-American.

Safar refused to be baited into such arguments. He repeatedly tried to sell the mayor on a citywide version of Freedom House as both the better, and cheaper, option. He pointed out that the cops made about fourteen grand a year to the medics' nine, and also that the police wagons were about twice as expensive as the ambulances Freedom House drove. When you tallied it all up, Safar said, it would cost the city just $2 per person for Freedom House to serve every corner of Pittsburgh. Still, his requests to expand were repeatedly denied. This left him with a simple, unanswered question—wasn't a life worth two dollars?

CHAPTER TWENTY-FOUR

Down at the base station, John was focused on the reality, not the politics of his job, and so if you asked him why all this was happening, he would've said he didn't know or even care, that he had a job to do, and the rest—all the fighting over budgets and territory and who did or didn't have the right to run an ambulance service in Pittsburgh—was just details. But when your life raft has sprung a leak and the water begins to rise, the details have a way of flooding in. Unable to block it all out and simply do their job, the medics slowly became aware of the city's opposition to their work and more specifically its opposition to *them*. They had some theories of their own about what it all meant.

Nobody actually believed the mayor was resisting their growth out of a distaste for public-private partnerships. His repeated refusal to absorb Freedom House and turn it into a city-run enterprise made this as baseless as any other of the justifications printed in the press. What did seem possible was that it was a calculated political move. It hadn't escaped John's attention, as the fighting dragged on into January and beyond, that 1973 was an election year. The mayor had begun his tenure by firing the long-serving and deeply entrenched police superintendent, then disbanded the heavy-handed police tactical squads that were so unpopular in the Black community, and further antagonized the city's cops by attempting to integrate precincts in majority Black neighborhoods. Handing ambulance operations to Freedom House would possibly cost a hundred twenty cops their jobs, and whether the powerful voting bloc of the police union would've forgiven him for that remained seriously in doubt.

Perhaps Flaherty knew this because for some time now his politics had been steadily drifting right, shoring up a part of his base that those early decisions alienated. He came out against school busing and opposed efforts to integrate a middle school. With this shift, he became so popular among the city's conservatives that he not only won the 1973 Democratic primary but also became a write-in candidate on the Republican ticket and won that too.

"The real tragedy about Peter is that he had the Blacks with him in the early days of his administration," the powerful state representative K. Leroy Irvis said at the time. "Now we have a jackass of a Mayor who seems only to play to the groundlings." Irvis, a Black lawmaker who represented the Hill, once considered Flaherty a friend, but now the two men were at odds. "His direction has been definitely anti-Black. As a private citizen, he has a right to his prejudices, but as a leader he can't be prejudiced."

Flaherty's about-face seemed part of a larger political shift, one that also lined up with the views of the man in the Oval Office. "It just ain't fashionable anymore to give money to Black organizations," said Bob Pitts, director of the Black Catholic Ministry in the Hill. Antipoverty programs from the '60s were drying up left and right. "Bein' Black ain't cool anymore. All you hear about us is that we're goin' around kickin' tail, raping ladies and boozin'." Phil Hallen tended to agree with this, believing Flaherty didn't like that Freedom House was a city program he couldn't control and, more specifically, that it was Black-owned and operated.

Maybe Hallen was wrong. Maybe Flaherty wasn't, as Phil often called him, "outright racist" but simply an opportunist, a guy who saw that the wave had crested and rolled back and aligned himself with the future. But maybe not.

Two things seemed to separate Pittsburgh from the other cities with advanced forms of street medicine. The first was that City Hall showed nothing but contempt for EMS here, in the town that arguably was its birthplace, while in cities like Miami, LA, and Columbus, medics were already considered a legitimate wing of public safety. The second difference, of course, was that in Pittsburgh the guys providing care were almost all Black, and whether or not you saw a connection between those two facts was probably a Rorschach for whether or not you considered yourself a part of the "silent majority." The guys at Freedom House did see the connection, and for them its reality meant living under a cloud of misunderstanding and suspicion. They understood instinctively that by refusing to embrace or legitimize them, the mayor emboldened the opposition to show a side of themselves normally kept hidden. It meant something as elemental as an emergency call—the simple act of saving a human life—could take on the dimensions of a disorienting, at times upside-down, unreality.

THE RED PHONE rang. Off they went. The ambulance racing through the Lower Hill with sirens wailing on its way to a woman, middle-aged, with chest pain in a high-rise. Outside John's window the Civic Center passed in a blur—they were crossing into downtown. John looked at George, who shrugged his shoulders, then reached down and flipped off the siren.

John shook his head. "This is stupid."

Up ahead the cars that a moment ago were pulling off to the right now hesitated. Brake lights flashed; drivers craned their necks to catch a glimpse of what was happening behind them—was the ambulance still coming? A few of them stayed to the right. Others kept going. Some stopped completely. John said it again—"This is stupid"—then eased the ambulance into the line of cars snaking its way into the city.

The invisible line separating the Hill from downtown was now the threshold at which an emergency vehicle carrying emergency medical technicians on their way to an emergency situation had to begin operating in all ways nonemergent. No more sirens downtown. This was something new. Hunt first raised the idea, but Flaherty made it law. The idea was to stop Freedom House's "reckless driving of ambulances," which they claimed not only imperiled drivers and pedestrians but also disrupted the business community. Hunt was helpful enough to suggest that Freedom House could, if it wanted, equip its ambulances with a little bell that paramedics might ring on their way to calls. The ban, of course, didn't apply to the cops speeding around town.

Pause here for just a moment and remember that by this time Freedom House had been surviving on half its originally promised operating budget for nearly four years. That because of the mayor's indifference or obstinance (or worse) it had missed out on millions—*millions*—in federal funding. That during this time it had continued to grow. New territory, new medics, new capabilities. What all this meant was that some need, somewhere, had to go unaddressed, and that need, as it turned out, was ambulance maintenance.

Freedom House had a fleet of five Chevy G20 vans. State of the art for the time, but that time was the '70s. The vans had heat, but it came out at one speed—*whoosh*. They had no air conditioning or power steering or antilock brakes. Turning took both hands, and forget about parking. Or stopping. They saw a lot of action, and the trim was always falling off, leaving in its wake a lonely trail of missing rivets. Don't even ask about hubcaps.

Crank the engine, and the grill—usually punched-in—got hot to the touch. They were loud, too. The rumble of a machine forty thousand miles past its prime, the high whine of four bald whitewall tires screaming against the pavement. Mechanical issues piled up. The door fell off Unit 2. Then its brakes failed. Then its rear window fell out. The steering on Unit 5 locked up. Unit 3 was maybe the worst—first its passenger seat came loose and tumbled over (with a passenger in it); then its engine caught fire (while driving).

Point is, just turning the key was an act of faith, and so to be rushing to an emergency—shoulders tired from wrestling a van without power steering, sweaty from the heat (and maybe an engine fire)—only to be forced, at an arbitrarily drawn boundary, to turn off your lights and sirens and slip back into midday traffic was almost more than anyone could bear. But they did bear it. Every day. With grace.

Still, if the city's plan was to make it difficult for Freedom House to operate by tossing up barriers that made the service seem less effective, then the plan was working. While John could have ignored it before, now it was affecting his ability to do his job. It felt to him as if the rug was being pulled out from under them, and that was frustrating and infuriating and incredibly sad in its own way, but that was just emotion talking, and emotion clouded your judgment when what the scene of an emergency called for was focus, so he channeled all that emotion into a hardened resolve. Whatever they threw in his way, he'd get over it and save the life at hand.

George pointed out the building. John eased the ambulance alongside the curb, put it in park. They were here, and none of the other stuff mattered. Just breathe it in, breathe it out. There was only the job.

Together, they packed their gear—oxygen, jump bag, cardiac monitor, and drug box—on the foldable stair chair and went inside. Through the lobby, into the elevator, gear jostling all the way up to the top, breathing stuffy air with the reception on the radio fading in and out, then *ding* and the doors opened. Down a hushed, carpeted hall and into a small office. Their patient sat in a chair. At the sound of an ambulance crew approaching, her eyes filled with the anticipation of help on the way. They flattened out to nothing when she saw the help was Black.

Here's where things get complicated. Running calls downtown where there were stores and businesses, entire blocks, without a single Black face meant that each ring of the red emergency phone raised the specter that the person on the other end of the line was white. This woman having chest pain at the end of a carpeted hall in a high-rise was white. But George just walked in and started talking like usual, making himself right at home. John was thinking his way through all the possible life threats hiding behind the symptoms, the treatment algorithms to deal with them, the drugs, and which hospital to go to. He was already kneeling by the woman's side when he really looked into her eyes for the first time and realized something was wrong. He started to explain chest pain and heart attacks, the diagnostic capabilities of the EKG machine at his side and the imperative of the next step, which was to unbutton her blouse so he could place the monitor's electrodes on her skin. She started shaking her head. He wasn't going to touch her, certainly not on her chest, and there definitely would be no unbuttoning of any blouses at all.

Her eyes flicked from John to George and back.

Maybe she was just unsettled. Chest pains are said to be accompanied by a sense of impending doom. But then it's possible, too, she'd heard the rumors that Freedom House wasn't just moving patients around the city but moving drugs as well. Whatever you wanted they had it, and when they weren't selling drugs, which probably was most of the time, they were running dice games. Nobody knew who started the rumors, but John speculated it was someone at City Hall, and he wasn't the only one. Crazy as they sounded, the rumors wouldn't die. They fed into stereotypes that were alive and well in the early '70s, and from those stereotypes it was only a short leap to believing they weren't just practicing medicine in the back of those ambulances, they were doing the unthinkable. And now here they were, as expected, trying to take her shirt off.

"Do you really have to do this?" She was shaking her head. "I would prefer you not do this. Can't we just go to the hospital?"

John's an optimist by nature. Every call had one purpose (to help) and a single outcome (a patient treated) so every time this happened, and it happened a lot, he would fail to see it coming. Certain things he expected. A degree of ignorance, maybe. What was a paramedic to a world that'd never heard of one? Just the week before there'd been a diabetic found down in a flophouse by his brother. The place was filthy and without furniture, and instead of plumbing there was a bucket next to the mattress. All the windows were painted shut, so the heat cooked that smell into everything. John and George were on the floor with him, their gear spread around them in an archipelago of medical know-how, when the brother stormed in.

"What the hell are you doing?!"

This happened sometimes. People accustomed to the sort of help that turned up in a police wagon expected the medics to arrive and disappear in a blur.

"I called you to take my brother to the hospital, and you're in here pissing around with him!"

Orderly, pensive John—sliding his glasses back into place—looked up to speak, to explain the intricacies of emergency medicine in general and paramedicine in particular. He didn't get past the first syllable. The man pointed a finger in his face. "If he dies . . . I'm coming after you."

The partners looked at each other—*Ready to go? Yeah, I think we should go*—and then they were scrambling. The gear and their patient, everything, hoisted over their shoulders as they ran for the door.

So sometimes there was confusion. But this wasn't confusion. It was uglier. It was disgust and hate. The woman, who may well have been having a heart attack, was physically recoiling in their presence. When all they wanted—the very reason she called them in the first place—was to help. John gave her the nicest smile he had.

"Without care you could die." He looked around the room. "And we're the only ones here to help. So, it's either us or . . ."

As in *either you let us do our job, or you could die right here on the floor of your office. Maybe make a mess of this nice carpet. But hey, at least you won't be sullied by a pair of handsy Black dudes.*

Ultimately, she consented to treatment and let John put on the EKG electrodes so he could get a reading on her heart and decide how best to treat her. That there was even a pause between the possibility that she might not make it and the reality of his hands on her skin more or less says it all. It happened again and again. In other high-rises, in houses. It happened in restaurants and on the street. After one particularly bad wreck, John had to plead with a woman to allow him to stabilize her broken femur with a traction splint because it would first require him to lift her skirt.

For many of John's patients, his arrival constituted a rare and uncomfortable interaction with Black people. The phenomenon of White Flight—significant enough here to have caused, by the mid-'70s, an overall drop in the city's population—carried white exiles from Pittsburgh proper to its outlying suburbs. Black families attempting to join them often faced resistance. In some of these suburbs the very idea of Black neighbors was considered odious enough that in at least one, Long Vue Manor on the east side, white homeowners were reportedly settling old grievances by "spite selling" their houses to Black families.

These white people may have lived in the suburbs, but they worked downtown. How someone who considered Black neighbors the ultimate punishment would perceive or treat John as he tried to help didn't dominate his thoughts—he was there to do a job.

But.

And this was a big but.

The cops.

Patients were one thing. They could be reluctant or even unwilling or flat-out difficult, but rarely were they a threat. The police were something else entirely.

WHEN JOHN LEAPT from the ambulance and ran across Centre Avenue toward the scene of the accident, his brain a whirling kaleidoscope of traumatic actions and their equal and opposite medical reactions, the one thing he didn't count on was being told to get the fuck out. But then again, the cops were already there when he arrived, and interactions between Freedom House and the police tended to get heated—even when what they were interacting over was a critically injured man.

Not even fifteen minutes earlier, this man, their patient, had been racing his car through the Hill, the world outside his window a blur of vacant lots and corner stores all hung with posters of Malcom X and Martin Luther King so faded by time they were barely legible. Just the year before, in 1972, the Beetle had finally beaten out the Model T to become the best-selling car of all time, so it's as likely as anything that this is what he was driving. Somewhere around the intersection of Centre and Crawford—maybe he lost control or maybe he was distracted or angry or simply didn't see it—he smashed head-on into a utility pole. The car crumpled.

Someone saw the accident and ran to call for help, starting the relay that led to Freedom House's red phone and then to John and George, who were only a few blocks away at Mercy Hospital. They jumped into their truck. A Pittsburgh police wagon was even closer and got there first. The cops hopped out, pried open the dented driver's side door, and started trying to drag the patient out. It was at this moment—the choke point between injury and treatment—that John and George arrived. John noticed first the obvious, that the Beetle was destroyed. Engine compartment caved in, windshield shattered, steering wheel bent. Safar had taught his medics kinesiology. They understood how the mechanics of a violent collision acted on the anatomy, how the organs traveled inside the body just as the body traveled inside the car, and how when the outside was stopped by smashing into something hard, the insides kept going until they too smashed against something hard. There's never one impact but many, and at this wreck they all suggested the very real possibility of serious injury.

So John started looking for the patient and found him—unconscious and stuck behind the wheel, flopping like a fish on a line as the cops tried frantically to yank him out. John jumped out of the ambulance and ran toward them shouting.

"No! No, no, no, no, no!"

He was worried about head injuries and internal bleeding but also the possibility of a spinal fracture. Speaking in support of the type of advanced medicine Freedom House practiced, county coroner Cyril Wecht would later tell the press "a person with a damaged spinal cord could become a quadriplegic if he is improperly handled." At this time, proper handling would've meant carefully removing the patient from his car and placing him on a long backboard with a rigid collar to keep his neck in line. Today the backboard's no longer used—that's how it works; medicine changes—but in 1973, it was the only acceptable way to move someone with a suspected spinal injury. And so when John saw that the man was limp, head flopping, as the cops dragged him out without a board or a collar or seemingly any regard at all for his ability to move his limbs in the future, he lost it.

"You can't do that! Don't do that!"

It was humid and hot, especially here in the street with the sun beating down. John was sweating, his heart pounding. He was out of breath and had nearly reached the cops when—

"Get the fuck out of here!"

It was so angry and violent, so sudden, John immediately stopped.

"You want me to put your ass in jail?"

John stood frozen. The road was slick with motor oil. The cop squared up, as if daring him to do something. John had seen officers use their nightsticks. He'd seen them bring their blackjacks down on someone's head so hard that the leather burst. He held his hands up. Took a step back. Broken bits of glass crunched under his boots.

"Okay. Okay."

The cop turned, and together with his partner they yanked the patient out and tossed him on their cot. They shoved him in the back of their wagon, slammed the doors, climbed up front, and sped away. John remained in the street, bystanders all around him, the mangled hulk of the VW Beetle slowly dying beside him. This was a low point. His ambulance and equipment, all that training, it felt completely useless. What was he even doing here?

George was already back in the ambulance. John joined him. People stared as they drove off empty-handed. It was frustrating and embarrassing, but it wasn't surprising. Not entirely.

IT WAS DESTINED to be this way from the start. All the way back in 1967, when the police decided not to support the creation of an ambulance service—that moment set the tone for how they would (or wouldn't) work with Freedom House. The paramedics would be a threat to their jobs and their turf, and the distrust that formed between them hadn't eased up one bit since. It was a clash of styles and mindset, of training, expertise, cultures—everything. The cops were focused on clearing obstructions and chaos, getting traffic flowing again. There was no thought of treating patients, of dragging out equipment and medicine and making a meal out of something that was, in their minds, all about velocity.

Mitch Brown explained the difference like this: "When Freedom House goes someplace, we're going there for one purpose. We're going to help the injured party." Obviously, on top of medicine, the cops had another job entirely—being cops.

Whenever John encountered pushback from the cops about treating a patient on the scene, and often enough he did, he tried to talk his way through it, to explain the emerging science and how it led to a new form of medicine that could save lives, and wasn't saving lives more important than the free flow of traffic? The other medics told him to let it go. They'd all seen things that would straighten your hair, but that's just how it was. Eugene Key said he once saw a cop drawing a chalk outline around a guy lying on the street. Cops did this with someone killed in a shooting or a stabbing or a wreck, so that even after the body was gone, investigators could piece together the crime scene and figure out what happened. But this man was still alive. Key pointed this out, but the cop just shrugged. "Yeah," he said, "but not for long."

Jules Brown, another medic, said it was a consequence of putting a rough mindset to fragile use. "The police are trained to be hard, that's their job. What if a cop is sent to pick up an injured man he's arrested before? What will go through the man's mind when the cop approaches? He'll think the cop is going to bash his head in like he did before."

The animosity went beyond the philosophical. This wasn't just a glaring difference of opinion and practice between competing ambulance services. In places like the Hill and Oakland, it touched every facet of their lives, and it went way back. Everyone knew the flashpoints. August 1968: two dozen Black men attacked Assistant Police Superintendent John Kelly during a heated city council meeting about the use of police tactical squads to break up demonstrations in Homewood. April 1970: more than four hundred police officers walked off the job to protest plans to diversify units patrolling majority-Black neighborhoods. Fall 1972: a young Black man was shot by police in a case of mistaken identity.

That members of the Pittsburgh police were at war with their own community was so apparent a US district court judge would eventually issue an injunction against a group of officers who, during the late '60s and early '70s, routinely stopped residents without cause, beat people who weren't committing crimes, used excessive force during arrests, harassed and intimidated residents, and conducted unlawful searches and seizures. Harvey Adams, one of the city's Black cops, alleged that his fellow officers would "abuse anyone who dared challenge their authority." Louis Mason, the city's first Black city council president, described the police as "too ingrained with racism to change." To wit: at a meeting to elect union delegates for the Fraternal Order of Police, a white cop running for office turned to a Black coworker and said, "Hey n—, you gonna vote for me?" An apology was issued, but the white cop still won his election.

It's impossible to imagine how, in such an environment, John or George or any other medic could do anything to stop a police officer from doing whatever he pleased on the scene of an emergency, even if what he was doing posed a direct threat to their patient. And this wasn't an accident or circumstance, but the direct result of the city's unyielding resistance to Freedom House at every turn. The people at the top abused them, and it normalized the behavior and all but ensured the abuse would trickle down into every interaction the medics had. Large or small. It sent out a signal that whatever they did, the pressure would never relent.

Each of these collisions registered and was recorded, like seismic vibrations on John's personal Richter scale, and over time they left cracks and fissures beneath the surface. But what was he or any of the medics to do? The only thing they could do. Same thing they always did. They slipped on their uniforms, drove to Presby, pounded out a handshake—one slow fist thumped atop the other—then fanned out across the Hill and saved lives.

To hell with everyone else.

CHAPTER TWENTY-FIVE

Picture a city teeming with people. The grit and glamour, the excitement, the crime, noise and energy, that frenzied rush of life. Then freeze it right there. Mid-stride. All those people, old, young, and in-between, the workers, the students, the infirm, those just this second being born. They look still on the outside, but beneath the surface each one is a thrumming instrument, carefully calibrated like the inner workings of a massive clock set to keep time with the universe itself. Hearts pounding sixty, eighty, a hundred times every minute, synapses firing exponentially faster. Oxygen rushing in and squeezing out with every breath. Blood coursing through their arteries, oozing all the way down to the capillaries before leaking, spent, into the veins, where it collects in the vena cava—the vasculature's central drain—to run straight back up into the chest, where it's swished through the heart and spat back out again, all the while carrying oxygen and sugar, sodium, calcium, potassium, feeding the cells, regrowing the cells, allowing them to contract and relax. To live. A dizzyingly complicated and terrifyingly fragile machine protecting and defining all we classify as a human life.

Now unfreeze them and watch. Off they go, the entire half million racing at breakneck speeds. In cars and on trains, at factories, steel mills, construction sites, coke barges, on bikes and skateboards, taking the steps two at a time. They're practically flying. Some of them actually are flying. And all around them are hard surfaces and sharp edges, paved roads and great heights, blast furnaces, two-ton trucks, toxic chemicals, flammable liquids, things to get cut on or choke on or make them explode. Dangers everywhere, and these hundreds of thousands of people are moving at incredible speeds, living their lives heedless of the danger. It would be so easy for any of it to break down or misfire or slip. To explode.

So easy in fact that it happens every day. All day long. People get hurt: they get cut, shot, run over, and burned. They're left bleeding and broken and clinically dead. And in 1970s Pittsburgh, when they needed help, Freedom House was there. Paramedics waiting in the little glass-walled base station at Presby, just outside the emergency department near the sliding double doors that let in a frozen burst of winter air every time they opened. Or maybe they were sitting out by the picnic table smoking cigarettes. Or grabbing lunch. Wherever they were, they were waiting. And as 1973 flipped over into 1974, George McCary and Bill Raynovich, Walt Brown, Dave Rayzer, Ron Ragin—they were all there, waiting to slip out beyond the wire to snatch life back from the edge of death. They'd been drawn together, this pack of rescuers, from every walk of life to ride out into the night, apostles of street medicine's greatest advance. They arrived as searchers—for a job after the service, to make their mother proud or prove their grandmother wrong. John came in search of a way to make something of himself, to become someone the world would have to reckon with, someone in control of his own life. And he found that at Freedom House. In rescuing others, he'd found a way to rescue himself.

A CRISP FALL day. Leaves changing, clouds softening into dollops of white in a gentle blue sky. The smell of charcoal and grilled sausage floating on the breeze as fifty-six thousand Pittsburghers crowded together at Pitt Stadium in the heart of Oakland to watch the Pitt Panthers play the William and Mary Tribe. At some point during the game the cheers and screams of the football fans were joined by a panicked cry for help. A sixty-eight-year-old man collapsed in the stands and went into cardiac arrest. His skin a deathly white, his eyes open and vacant. Then sirens and a commotion as two medics in white Freedom House jackets ran up the stairs. One started CPR, while the other switched on their cardiac monitor, ripped the man's shirt open, and then placed paddles on his chest. "Clear!" With an electric pop his body arced and bounced off the ground. His heart started beating. The crowd, jittery with adrenaline and fear and gratitude, cheered as they left for the hospital.

Days, maybe weeks, or months later—it all blends. Late afternoon, Centre Avenue. A twenty-five-year-old man threw a television out of his open window and down onto the street below. An explosion of electronic miscellany. The cops arrived, and over the next four hours the young man, short and muscular, with a shaved head and a polka-dot shirt, repeatedly leaned from his window to yell at the police. There were a handful of small flowerpots on the windowsill, some filled with tiny cacti, and at one point, as he came and went, barricaded in his apartment, he threw one down and hit a cop. The show was over, the police were going in, and Freedom House was called out for the inevitable transport. Just after nine p.m., the cops broke down his door and rushed inside. The medics followed them in. They emerged a few minutes later with the man on their stretcher. The polka-dot shirt was gone, but he now had a towel over his head and shouted, "He got a yellow Cadillac!" As is so often the case with an ambulance service that spends its days crawling over every inch of a city, they knew this man and remembered that just a few months before, he was hit by a car and suffered a head injury, the result of which, according to his neighbors, was that he sometimes sat on the stoop or up above in his window to "yell at motorists or pedestrians or nobody at all." He was loaded into the ambulance and, rather than sent to jail, transported to Western Psych.

Also that fall, an eighty-one-year-old woman lay half-awake, smoking in bed. She lived in a three-story wooden rooming house, and as she drifted off to sleep, the cigarette slipped from her fingers. The house was at peace until half past two, when the calm was broken by the screams of the landlord running through the halls shouting, "Fire!" One at a time, doors opened as people poked their heads out to find the halls full of smoke. Flames followed, and within minutes the building was engulfed in what would become a three-alarm blaze. In the rush to get out, people got desperate. A child was tossed from a third-floor window and caught by a security guard on the street. The woman whose cigarette started the fire was dead—she'd be found later, spread flat across her bed—and seven others were injured. But there were no local ambulances available to help them. This rooming house wasn't in the Hill or Oakland; it was north of the Allegheny River. Nevertheless, Freedom House responded. All afternoon long, orange and white ambulances transported the burned and traumatized across the river to the hospital.

Another call that season, this one downtown. Inside the hushed security of a bank. The manager had a heart attack, and there was Freedom House, creeping along (siren-free) to treat the patient and calm the crowd, leaving everyone marveling at "how lucky" they were to have such a program in the city.

Medics were dragged back into the classroom, this time to teach emergency medicine to future doctors at the Pitt medical school. Day after day, call upon call—so many that they overlapped and melted together—Freedom House defied the mayor, keeping this city in motion from falling apart, and existed as a potent symbol of ingenuity and perseverance, of the absurdity of intolerance, the face of medicine in all its changing hues, but first, and most importantly, the gently raised voice of a forgotten neighborhood. The world was taking notice.

BOOK FOUR

CHAPTER TWENTY-SIX

Nancy Caroline was working in the Presby ICU the night it all started. She was partway through a shift and perfectly attuned to the slightest variation in the wheezing ventilators, the errant ping of a monitor but completely unaware that Safar and his ambulances were about to change the entire course of her life, that people she'd never heard of, like John Moon and Walt Brown, and even some she had heard of, like Pete Flaherty, were set to scramble and recast everything she thought was important. It was late on the night of November 11, 1974. The ICU was dark and quiet, almost somber, matching the weather and also, increasingly, Nancy's mood. At some point, as she wandered among the sleeping patients, checking charts and monitors and lab values, placing central lines or reviewing the occasional scrip, a trio of doctors walked in. She recognized only one: Sol Edelstein.

"Dr. Safar has a . . . job for you," he said.

No question, this was weird. It was awfully late at night for them to wander in, and anyway last time Nancy checked she was three months into a difficult and exacting critical care fellowship. She might've been brand new and fairly inexperienced, but she was pretty certain about one thing: "I already have a job."

Edelstein's smile suggested maybe Nancy wasn't being ordered to do whatever Safar had in mind, but she wasn't exactly being asked either.

"Dr. Safar would like you to be the medical director for Freedom House."

She wrinkled her brow. "What's Freedom House?"

"It's a group of EMTs."

"What's an EMT?"

"Someone who works on an ambulance."

"I've never been on an ambulance."

"It can be arranged," Edelstein said, growing impatient. Another of the doctors jumped in. "You'll love it. Once you get used to it."

That also struck Nancy as strange, but there was too much happening at once to parse it all. "Why me?"

"Because no one else—"

"Because," Edelstein cut in, "Dr. Safar felt you'd be the most competent person for the job."

Nancy crossed her arms, leaned back into a posture of wild skepticism. "I've only met him once, for two minutes, on the street. He said hello, I said hello, and that was it. How come he thinks I'm so special?"

Edelstein, an anesthesiologist around the same age as Nancy, fixed her with a calm stare. "Nancy." The patient, indulgent voice of a doctor prescribing a long and difficult treatment. "Scan this material Dr. Safar sent. Think it over."

He handed her a thick stack of files, articles, notes, and scribbles—the accumulated miscellanea of seven frustrating years. Edelstein suggested she take her time. Safar didn't need an answer until Wednesday. Nancy looked up.

"That's the day after tomorrow!"

"So it is."

As they turned to leave, one of the doctors she hadn't met looked over his shoulder and said, "You'll really love it."

Then the door shut, and it was quiet again.

Later that night, Nancy found a hidden corner and dug into the files. What she read was a confounding story of challenges and complications, of racism, financial troubles, and an organization holding on by its fingertips. It was a window onto a world stretching back nearly a decade, yet there seemed to be a new urgency, some desperate push to tie up loose ends that the documents made clear had been dangling since 1966 and to the question of "Why me?" she scribbled a second question, a sort of companion to the first—"Why now?"

THE ANSWER WAS mainly that 1974 had been a big year in America, around the world, and even closer to home. Everywhere things were happening. Stephen King's *Carrie*, the Rumble in the Jungle, the fifty-five-mile-per-hour speed limit. Richard Nixon resigned the presidency. In such a climate, maybe nobody was paying much attention to western Pennsylvania, but things were churning there, and in Pittsburgh, 1974 was the year Peter Flaherty abruptly changed his mind about ambulances.

The news that the mayor had pulled a U-turn and was now prepared to bring the city's emergency services into the twentieth century came in March, but the wheels were set in motion months before, when the city council openly endorsed EMS and urged Flaherty to join them. He refused. In his 1974 budget proposal, the mayor made no provision whatsoever for upgrading the service. Frustrated, the council acted without him and in December 1973 approved a budget that included $550,000 to modernize ambulance care, effectively forcing the mayor's hand. Though Flaherty refused to sign it, the budget passed anyway. With more than half a million dollars earmarked to upgrade EMS, it seemed this year the ambulance question would finally be answered.

But nobody knew when. January came and went, and so did February, and still Flaherty refused even to acknowledge the money. March broke cold and damp the way it always does, and it seemed nothing would happen then, either, until, suddenly, on the eleventh, Police Superintendent Colville walked into council chambers and announced plans to buy five specialized ambulances, plus equipment to upgrade the city's existing fleet. In addition, the hundred cops currently manning the city's police wagons would be put through a training course so that when all this new gear arrived, they'd know how to use it. Nowhere in his announcement did he mention that these specialized ambulances and advanced training might not be available if it hadn't been for Freedom House. In fact, he didn't mention Freedom House at all. Colville concluded by speculating it would take six months for all this equipment and the city's newly trained cops to hit the streets.

Flaherty's turnabout was sudden. As recently as December, he'd insisted that expanding city ambulance service "would be a mistake," leading Councilman Robert Rade Stone to question why Flaherty had now chosen in March to pursue an advanced ambulance service. "Whether his present aspirations for higher and better things have broadened his thinking, I do not know," Stone said, referring to Flaherty's recently announced candidacy for US Senate. "But we welcome his change of heart." Still, Stone was frustrated that Flaherty had dragged his feet so long. "That the Mayor did not see the wisdom of this program in December is amazing."

Even more amazing was his plan to disband Freedom House. Flaherty wanted only police in his ambulance corps, which meant the city would cancel the contract with Freedom House, effectively abandoning its thirty-five medics. That they were already better educated and more experienced than the cops would be, even after their new training course, seemed not to matter. Opponents of this plan could find no logic in its course. They rose up in defiance.

Press conferences were held in support of Freedom House by activists both Black and white, who stood before microphones dressed in classically '70s clothes—lots of buttons and colors and splashy prints, mustaches, big collars, bigger hair. They came from all over. The NAACP, the Hill House, Women in the Urban Crisis, Council of Catholic Women, Catholic Interracial Council, the Thomas Merton Center, Pittsburgh Plan, Allegheny Residents Council, the Goodwill Association, Youth City. They were full-throated in their support of

Freedom House and had plenty to say about the mayor's plan. State Representative Irvis: "Freedom House would be replaced by an inferior grade of ambulance care." Elizabeth Wolfskill of the Western Pennsylvania Coalition for Human Needs: "It is foolish and insulting to Pittsburghers [that] $500,000 has suddenly been allocated to the Bureau of Police for ambulance training and equipment, when an existing and proven emergency ambulance service could be continued and expanded." Her organization lobbied the city to give the entire amount to Freedom House.

Even the *Pittsburgh Post-Gazette*, which wasn't exactly liberal (it published daily Bible verses), came out against the plan on its editorial page. Given how little trust the Black community had in the cops, the paper questioned the wisdom of putting police in charge of their emergency medical care, suggesting instead that Freedom House be expanded. After all, the *Post-Gazette* noted, the only reason Pittsburgh was paying to upgrade its ambulance system at all was that Freedom House had demonstrated just how bad the police service really was.

As everyone around him was fighting over his future, John did his best to carry on. Anything happening in City Hall, even efforts ostensibly made in his defense, he viewed as background noise. He was too consumed by the day-to-day realities to consider long-term conjecture. Besides, things were busier now at home. His son, John, was five, and Betty was pregnant, this time with a daughter the couple would name Adrienne. If the job generated any concerns at all, for John they were those of a parent. Shortly after Adrienne was born, he was dispatched to an unresponsive baby. He arrived in the middle of the night to find the child not breathing, classic presentation of Sudden Infant Death Syndrome. She was the same age as his own daughter, three months, and when he lifted her from the crib, she was cold. John kept his composure on the scene, but the moment he cleared the call, he punched out and went home. He woke Adrienne from a sound sleep and held her for two hours just to feel her warmth.

But not everyone was able to tune out the noise. If the police retook EMS in the Hill, several medics told the press they would go back to school to further their medical education, while others said they might have to leave medicine altogether. Overall, however, their biggest concern was for their patients. "If a guy has OD'd or flipped out," Jules Brown told the *Pittsburgh Post-Gazette*, "as soon as they see that badge there's going to be hostility and it's going to be a bad situation."

Mitch Brown, as ever, was outspoken on the issue. "We have expert emergency medical care. The police department does not," he told the press. "I know of nowhere in the United States that police are providing the kind of care we provide." Then, more provocatively: "How would you like to receive emergency medical attention from a policeman with a stethoscope around his neck and a gun on his hip? The old shoot and patch-up theory."

Ordinary citizens also came forward. Sidney Feiler, vice principal of Fifth Avenue High School, wrote an op-ed praising the Freedom House medics for their unstinting professionalism. When called, she said they arrived "unfailingly and almost immediately," with a "high degree of efficiency and effectiveness." Their presence, she said, made everyone feel more secure. Removing the medics would be "unconscionable." Another bewildered resident asked what seemed the essential question: "Why should the police, already burdened with law enforcement duties, be given the enormous task of upgrading emergency care when a competent agency geared to do that already exists?"

This question wasn't purely rhetorical—budget constraints had kept the police department from filling vacancies for three years, leaving the department short roughly four hundred officers—but the mayor failed to mount a convincing argument. As spring turned to summer the question rose time and again: Why not Freedom House?

It was a good question, but maybe not as simple as it seemed. By mid-'74, in the upside-down world Freedom House had been living in, this question had somehow become the central issue facing the service and, at the same time, almost entirely irrelevant. Fact is, Freedom House was on the brink of collapse. In July, the federal grant that paid much of their expenses was set to expire, and no provision had been made by the city to make up for the lost revenue. Bills were stacking up, and whether or not Freedom House would continue to exist, let alone expand, was very much in doubt.

When he heard this news, Flaherty shrugged it off. Under his plan Freedom House would be replaced by the cops anyway. What did it matter if it happened in July or sometime later when the police were ready to take over? This begged the obvious question of who would cover emergencies in their absence, but this too was waved off. Police Superintendent Colville personally didn't see a problem with a gap in coverage, since the area in question was only a small (Black) portion of the city.

Not everyone at City Hall was so indifferent. Councilman Stone observed: "It would be the height of irony if this organization created to save lives in an emergency situation should be itself incapable of saving its own life." The *Pittsburgh Post-Gazette* called the very idea "short-sighted." Tim Stevens, executive director of the NAACP, went much further, calling it "a pattern of ripoff in Black programs in Pittsburgh and across the nation."

At an emergency council meeting to discuss the possibility of the city covering Freedom House's budgetary shortfall, Flaherty tried to remain noncommittal about the service's future. But his sanguine responses only made the assembled crowd angrier. He switched tactics. A mayor's job was hard, he said, full of difficult budget decisions, and he was trying to keep a lid on spending. This was a hard stance to defend. By now people had read the stories and knew that cops were paid significantly more than the medics and therefore were the more expensive of the two options. Clearly this wasn't a financial issue—the numbers simply didn't support the claim. When again Flaherty tried to wriggle free and explain, the crowd shouted him down. Their boos got so loud at times they had to be gaveled. The meeting ended without any concrete decisions, but it was clear Freedom House's supporters wouldn't stand by quietly and watch the service die.

Then, just a few weeks later, things got even hotter for the mayor as chaos spilled out into the city itself.

ON JULY 3, Pittsburgh police officer Patrick Wallace was shot and killed while making an arrest in the Pittsburgh neighborhood of Brushton. In the immediate aftermath of the shooting, the community's sympathy was firmly on the cops' side. The lead suspect had recently escaped from Western Penitentiary, and his accomplices were described by neighbors as "bad actors" who made everyone around them feel unsafe. But as the manhunt for the killer dragged on and intensified, that goodwill quickly curdled. Soon complaints of harsh and indiscriminate tactics began to surface.

One night, officers investigating the murder stopped two men on the Fort Duquesne Bridge. According to their complaint, one was handcuffed and beaten, while the other was elbowed in the face so hard he needed six stitches to close the wound. They also claimed one of the cops yelled, "I'll kill the n— that killed my brother!" Though the complaint didn't specifically identify who yelled this, Wallace's younger brother was on the force at the time.

On another occasion, police entered an apartment building and battered down twenty-four doors in response to a tip that the killer might have been hiding there. Many of the cops were in plainclothes and heavily armed when they arrived, firing tear gas into the halls before forcing residents from their homes. People stood outside for hours as the search dragged on and returned when it was over to find their doors knocked from the hinges. Asked about the behavior of his fellow officers, one cop was quoted as saying, "Things are tense, and they overreacted a bit."

State Attorney General Israel Packel ordered an investigation into allegations of police brutality, and angry residents picketed in front of

Flaherty's house to protest what they considered a brazen trampling of their rights.

Still the mayor held firm on plans to hand emergency medical services over to his embattled police department. Internally though, his plans were falling apart. Colville's statement back in the spring that all the training and equipping would be done within six months turned out to be hopelessly optimistic. The training, initially set to wrap in June, would now not be completed until August. The date was later pushed back even further, to December. The ambulances that were supposed to arrive in October hadn't even been ordered when October rolled around. They were now due to arrive in January, and with any luck they'd be on the road by February, more than a year after money was approved and months later than promised, but this too was wishful thinking, and officials close to the process speculated it would likely be even later than that.

By fall, everything was in disarray. Incomprehensible as it seemed, a city that for seven years was home to a modern, trendsetting, and incredibly competent ambulance corps somehow found itself in 1974 fumbling the effort to replace it with a service everyone already acknowledged to be inferior. Maddening. But perhaps not surprising.

"If this was mostly a white organization," paramedic Eugene Key speculated, "I don't think this would be happening."

Finally, it all became too much. With the pretense that this was an impartial decision based on economics and civics and medical know-how, on what was best for the city's five hundred thousand residents, crumbling under the weight of its own absurdity, Flaherty was forced to relent. He agreed to fund Freedom House for the rest of '74 and through 1975. What would happen beyond that, he refused to say. This last-second pardon was a sobering reminder that even after everything they'd accomplished, the mayor was willing to let the organization die an undignified and very public death. In the eyes of some people—people who mattered—they hadn't earned their place and maybe never would.

CHAPTER TWENTY-SEVEN

This was the last straw for Safar—at least for a moment. Years of fighting the city and the county while also running Freedom House and heading up the anesthesia department had worn him down. That summer he resigned from the board. Briefly. The moment he left, something came along to bring him back to Freedom House. In September, Safar was invited to join President Gerald Ford's five-member Interagency Committee on EMS, established to help direct federal ambulance policy. High on the group's list of priorities was a push to formalize EMS training. Though it wouldn't be announced until January, their recommendation would be to give a single ambulance service the honor of creating and field-testing what would become the nation's first standardized paramedic curriculum.

This would clearly be a huge boon for any service, but imagine what it might do for one already dangling by a thread. Though Safar never said this was why he returned, you don't have to connect many dots to assume it was. And just as surely, he would've known that whichever service ultimately was chosen to serve as a model for these new national training standards would, in effect, become *the* national standard for EMS services nationwide. This was exactly the sort of recognition and attention, the legitimacy, that just might permanently prevent an antagonistic mayor from shutting them down.

Safar desperately wanted Freedom House to be chosen.

THERE WAS ONLY one problem. The organization had become disorganized. Much of the blame lay at the feet of Flaherty and Hunt, but some of it Safar placed upon himself. Though he created and administered Freedom House's training program, once the service was up and running he'd been less than attentive. Aside from his other work obligations, he'd left for a year-long sabbatical in 1969. Plus, the doctor he appointed to serve as medical director—the physician charged with the day-to-day duty of updating and enforcing an EMS service's medical protocols—Don Benson, was called up for military service and later decided to leave the organization altogether. For several years the service had a series of temporary medical directors, all of them part-time and not heavily involved. Freedom House needed someone new at the helm.

They also needed an upgrade. If Freedom House was to be viewed as the best in the nation, they'd have to train and operate as the best in the nation. While they were off fighting for their lives, new tactics and equipment had come along, and a whole new understanding of emergency medicine had been born. Freedom House might have been the first, but others were pulling ahead. To catch up, additional training would be necessary. Included in all this, of course, was Safar's deep-rooted desire to right his failure with the inaugural training class in 1967. This time, the medics would master the art of intubation.

Pulling this off would require the direct, day-to-day leadership of a brilliant doctor. Someone young and fearless and energetic, someone who'd throw themselves into the role with passion and wisdom and a resolve to get the job done quickly. Safar carefully combed over his roster of physicians looking for just the right name, hoping to create a master list and from that a short list and from that an appointee. Instead, he came up with no one. He had nobody who fit the bill. Impressive, he had. Dynamic, too. Energetic, brilliant—sure. But none of them wanted the job. Oh, he asked. But his doctors were all busy with their fellowships and more than a little hesitant to distract themselves with a side project they neither understood nor appreciated.

Then there was all the fighting with City Hall, not to mention tensions between Presby and Freedom House, which had mellowed since the beginning but weren't entirely gone. Heap on top of all this the cultural gap a physician would have to bridge. Any doctor practicing medicine in '74 had entered med school in the '60s, and let's be honest, most people going through medical school in the 60s were both white and well-off and couldn't relate to the medics who were neither. Those he'd managed to snare never warmed up to the work. In early photos, physicians can be seen standing off to the side, at a remove from the staff they led.

Safar needed a doctor who was singular of vision, who possessed both the clinical detachment and dedication to medical advancement necessary to propel them over every obstacle in their path or else bulldoze right through it. In short, he needed a doctor like himself. But he couldn't find one. Instead, what his search yielded, almost accidentally, was Nancy Caroline—a thirty-one-year-old critical care fellow driven as much by passion and human connection as she was by science and who, on the night Sol Edelstein approached her in the ICU, was struggling every bit as much as the organization she would be asked to save.

CHAPTER TWENTY-EIGHT

Nancy was always of two minds. A teenage poet who worked part-time in the Mass General pathology department, a precocious student who very nearly dropped out of medical school, a storyteller and free spirit, a prankster, but also a scientific explorer. She was a feminist who fell into relationships with impossible men and then did the heavy lifting. Nancy understood from an early age she would leave a mark on the world and kept a careful record of her journey. She saved everything. In her correspondence, Nancy scribbled caustic asides and whirly sketches; she once drew two images of a heart: one as it actually looks in the body and the other as it looks only in popular culture. She was at once whimsy and precision and never tried to separate the two.

Nancy Caroline was born in June 1944, in the Boston suburb of Newton. Her father, Leo, ran a men's clothing store, and her mother, Zelda, would outlive her. She and her older brother, Peter, were raised Jewish and came from a long line of well-educated people who appeared in her carefully drawn family trees less as ancestors than as impressive collections of graduate degrees. Her pedigree was Ivy League—nine relatives attended Harvard alone. This was the legacy Nancy inherited, and she was determined to live up to it.

She wrote out daily schedules in military time—"0845 swimming; 1000 CHW; 1130 Collins; 1300 home"—and was named editor in chief of her high school paper. As always, there was a flipside to this. Responsibility's evil but much more endearing twin. She flushed the toilet one day while her brother was showering and then ran outside as he howled, tingling with the thrill of mischief and discovery. She convinced herself the trapdoor in the bathroom ceiling led not to the attic but beyond, to some exotic and adventurous world. The day she left home for college, Nancy dragged a ladder into the bathroom and climbed up to the trapdoor—just to see—but changed her mind at the last second. Maybe it was better to let it be, to leave the magic unpierced.

In the 1960s, when Harvard still admitted only men, intellectual, independent-minded women with their eyes on Cambridge applied to its sister school, Radcliffe College. So after she graduated from high school a year early, that's where Nancy went. She studied linguistics, quoted Camus, occasionally slipped into German, and helped support herself by ghost writing scientific articles for faculty members. In the spring of 1966—the year Safar's daughter and David Lawrence died, when the White Paper was published and the Highway Safety Act passed—just days before her twenty-second birthday, she graduated summa cum laude and then, naturally, took a year off.

She eventually decided on medical school and chose Case Western University in Ohio, which was something like medicine's answer to eccentricity. There were no grades or class rankings; students were given time for electives and, unusual among medical schools, put in position to treat patients their very first year. One man decided admissions: the Harvard-educated "Cactus Jack" Caughey, who was both intimidating and respected and once said of his students, "I try to care for [them] the way they'll care for their patients." Cactus Jack stamped Nancy with his seal of approval and sent her on to the pursuit that would define the rest of her life.

From the moment she cracked her first textbook, medicine became her path, but Nancy's creative, restless, churning mind strained even against Case Western's admittedly permissive boundaries. She wrote short fiction, poetry, and articles. She made a surrealist short film—because the '60s, because college. She nearly dropped out after her first year, but her uncle, a urologist, convinced her to stay. He told her about the money and the prestige and, knowing his audience, confided that being a doctor was "a badge of independence" that would keep her from ever having to answer to anyone else. So Nancy stayed. She graduated in 1971 with just over $1,000 in loans, then completed her residency at University Hospitals in Cleveland. From there it was off to Presby for a critical care fellowship under Safar.

When she hit Pittsburgh in 1974, Dr. Caroline rented a small apartment in a three-story brick building on a tree-lined street in Highland Park, on the east side of the city. Her cousin Audrey lived nearby. They hung out; they cooked; they shouted above the constant clang of radiator pipes that lined Nancy's walls. They were busy, tiring times. When not at home, she was in the ICU.

Nancy smoked a lot, too much by her own reckoning, and one afternoon she stepped outside the hospital for a cigarette. It was August, she'd barely just arrived, and as she leaned against the wall next to Sol Edelstein, another of Safar's fellows, a siren rose up in the distance. The sound got louder until it was no longer so distant, and as the ambulance roared past them, she asked Sol if any of the Presby doctors ever made ambulance runs. Here Edelstein got cagey. He shrugged, told her not to bother with it, that an ambulance was just an ambulance and whatever happened in there wasn't *medicine* medicine. And anyway, Edelstein told her, there was this whole thing between the service and the city and, well, it was a mess. Best to let it go. So she let it go. Nancy took one final drag, dropped her cigarette, crushed it out beneath her shoe, and forgot all about ambulances.

AND NOW, THREE months later, the ambulances found her. Nancy carefully stacked the papers she'd been given on Freedom House and set them aside. It was beyond late, the ICU beyond quiet. She smirked. So this was how she'd been "chosen." Because nobody else would take the job, because in an idle moment she'd asked Sol a question and, months later, he remembered it and passed it along to Safar, who was so desperate for a doctor to guide the ambulance service that her offhanded and innocent question (constituting the entirety of her qualifications) was deemed to be qualification enough. This hardly felt like an opportunity.

Still.

She was intrigued. It was different. It offered the possibility of fun, racing on an ambulance to who knows where. It was the trapdoor all over again—whatever lay on the far end of an ambulance run must surely be exotic and adventurous. And she didn't care that the other doctors had turned the job down, that they didn't think it was worth their time. Nancy was a born contrarian. Her brother, Peter, would tell you the surest way to get her to do something was to tell her not to do it.

The next day, she responded to Safar not with the yes he clearly expected from her—or even the apologetic please-no-I-don't-have-the-time-for-this evasion the other doctors had given. Nancy responded, characteristically, with questions. A whole barrage of them. Safar was in charge of her fellowship, the head of the anesthesiology department, the Father of CPR, more or less the inventor of the ICU, and yet she was writing to say he'd have to cough up a lot more information, plus a handful of assurances, before she'd even consider his request.

Safar must've smiled as he read her note. At last he'd found his doctor.

WHAT FOLLOWED WAS a negotiation. Nancy at first said no. She'd already failed her Internal Medicine Boards and had to prepare (seriously this time) for a retest the following spring. But Safar persisted. When he first accepted the Pittsburgh job back in 1960, it wasn't for the city, which he found polluted and old-fashioned, but to take on a challenge everyone warned him couldn't be done. Creating a robust anesthesiology department, a new specialty at the time, would require major change, and the Pitt University health system was considered by many too big for change. But a good fight was what drove him. He was so excited that he sold the Baltimore dream house he and Eva had designed before construction was even finished. He never even inquired about his salary; he just went. This impulsive leap might've perfectly illustrated Safar's unsentimental and relentless pursuit of what's next, but it in no way prepared him for how normal people might act under similar circumstances.

For most doctors, the seemingly impossible task of helping build a state-of-the-art anesthesiology department within a ponderous bureaucracy wasn't reason enough or even reason at all. They also balked at the pay and were hesitant to drop everything and relocate to a small city that didn't always create a great first impression. So Safar turned his energy up to eleven and moved mountains to get them excited. He wined and dined. He leaned heavily on Eva's remarkable charm and hospitality. He brought people in when the weather was at its best and the smog ringing the city was in ebb. And when all this failed, he pressed and pestered until, finally, worn down, they said yes. Safar eventually got so good at drawing people to him that his former colleagues back in Baltimore—his favorite poaching ground—started calling him the Pied Piper.

He now brought all of this experience to bear against Nancy. He promised to scale back her other duties, pay a good salary, and give her free hand to run things as she saw fit. He assured her the job would be part-time (it wasn't), that other critical care fellows would help (they didn't), and that the real work wouldn't begin until July (more like immediately). Over the next few weeks, he turned her no into a maybe and finally a yes. That winter Nancy traveled to Israel and while there, on December 17, she received her formal offer. Safar was triumphant—"1975 will be the year when the dream of 1969 will become realized"—but her peers less so. One wrote to assure her the job was "not as bad as it seems."

When Nancy returned to Pittsburgh, Freedom House occupied only the edges of her mind. Soon it would dominate everything.

CHAPTER TWENTY-NINE

January 1975 was a chaotic time in the base station. The medics had just emerged from their toughest year yet, a striking statement considering all the storms they'd endured over the previous six years, and they were about to learn that change was again on the horizon. One afternoon, John walked in to begin his shift. At some point among all the yelling and the laughing, the gusts of cold that crept through the sliding doors, Mitch Brown walked in with news and said for everyone to listen up.

"Now look, fellas, we got a new medical director who's really good, honest." By this point he'd known about Nancy for a week but had kept it to himself. Over in his chair in the corner, John listened. "I want you to treat her nicely."

If Brown was trying to sneak this last part through, it didn't work.

"Her?!"

Pandemonium. "Listen, fellas." Shouting over the noise: "Just give her a chance!"

Amid all the commotion, John slipped out. He'd give this woman a chance—what choice did he have, really? And anyway, he didn't figure she'd make much difference. Probably she'd be like the other doctors who'd come and gone, and she too would just come and go. She'd likely be present from a distance, there but mostly not. As he hopped into the ambulance, he put her out of his mind. He had a job to do, and this was above him, a decision handed down by Safar, and if she was good enough for *him*, then surely, if nothing else, she had her shit together.

ACROSS TOWN, NANCY sat huddled in her Highland Park apartment freezing. Turns out the radiators that clanged all night produced no heat. Smoke from the fireplace in the apartment below seeped into hers, blanketing everything in a haze. She hardly knew the dark city that lay beyond her windows and wasn't at all certain what she was doing there. Her Internal Medicine Boards were only a few months away, and to the stress of the exams she could now add the anxiety of a strange new job. Though she was technically in charge of them, truth was she still didn't know exactly what paramedics were or what they might expect of her.

Very quickly Nancy's (not so) part-time job became even less so. Safar wanted to put Freedom House on level ground with the highest performing systems in the country and developed an intense three-month course to get them there. Then he asked Nancy to teach it. Heightened stakes were added to her increasing workload in early January, when the president's Interagency Committee on EMS made public their recommendation that a standardized paramedic training course—which was ultimately to be administered by, and funded through, the Department of Transportation—be developed and one ambulance service be chosen to create it.

Her hiring, the urgency behind the course, and this announcement were not mere coincidences. Nancy's mandate was clear: revamp Freedom House, turn it into the obvious choice for this high-profile role, and, in the process, save the service from closure. Alone in her apartment, Nancy could feel the pressure mounting. Looking for guidance, she traveled to Miami and then Jacksonville, two cities operating on the outer edge of what was possible in an ambulance, in the hopes of getting her head around the task. It didn't help. In Miami she felt like an unwanted observer in a closed fraternity, and in Jacksonville she was told, "We try not to bring the colored trash to the good hospitals."

She returned to Pittsburgh every bit as lost as when she left. Her usual restlessness began to creep back in, though now it was compounded by the bleak Pennsylvania winter and an unshakeable sense of loneliness. In coming to Pittsburgh from Cleveland she'd left behind the man she loved.

THE AFFAIR STARTED in the sweltering summer of 1971. Nancy, twenty-seven, was in the earliest days of her residency. Manny, a forty-four-year-old doctor working in Cleveland whose full name was Manuel Soto Curiel, was married with three children back home in St. Louis. Things got serious very quickly. Manny felt they had to—if this wasn't love, how could he justify betraying his family? They spent all their time together. They went for walks and to the theatre. Nancy kept the ticket stubs. Eventually, he moved on again, this time to Boston. She moved to Pittsburgh but daydreamed of being with him on the banks of the Charles River. She helped manage his affairs from afar, the girlfriend as secretary. *I am writing on behalf of. . . .*

Nancy worked endlessly to keep the distance from pulling them apart. She sent cards, pictures, and books. She signed her letters "Your SLT" (Stupid Little Thing). She wrote a poem in stanzas that slanted across the page, her conflicting and complicated feelings wrapped up in a refrain that asked, over and over, *Will you dive after me if I sink too deep?*

Over the next few months, this unanswered question grew and consumed her. All was not well.

Manny drank; he suffered bouts of depression; he disappeared for "lost weekends," returning to accuse Nancy of pushing him away. She carried a heavy, lovesick feeling through the fall of 1974 and into the winter that she hoped to shake, or at least relieve, during her visit to Israel. And briefly she did. But the warmth of those days quickly faded once she returned to Pittsburgh. Her relationship was faltering, and as she often did, she felt an emptiness that work or study alone could not fill. "Rain the interminable," she wrote. "The endless gray saps my energies, replacing them with a restlessness akin to longing, but without an objective."

Radcliffe, med school, residency. Years of hard work and the faithful dedication to a man who was slowly unwinding—she'd been relentless, selfless, and it brought her here. To an empty apartment and a job she could barely fathom. She needed an escape from the painful unraveling of her relationship, from the cold, from the loneliness. She wrote of "waiting for meaning to overtake my existence." Nancy wanted "a new life," "a cause, perhaps. Some all-consuming purpose in which to channel a thousand scattered energies."

What she got was Freedom House.

CHAPTER THIRTY

Things did not start well. Nancy's first memorable interaction with her new charges came just days into the job, when the Freedom House crew chiefs, three "very imposing, bearded, machismo characters" whom she'd never met, barged into her office to air their grievances. She had no idea what they were talking about—their problems, much like the job itself, were foreign to her—but she wasn't going to admit that. Not to them. She smiled and nodded while they spoke and, the moment they were gone, shut the door and sank into her chair. Whatever this thing was that she'd gotten herself into, it had arrived in full force. She was a young doctor who'd only recently completed her residency, placed in charge of a corps of paramedics whose training and scope of practice, potential, limitations—in some cases even their very existence—was almost entirely unknown to physicians boasting a lifetime of experience. She'd very quickly jumped in the deep end, and there was nothing to do now but swim.

For the next week, Nancy barricaded herself behind a wall of work. Day and night she listened in over the radio, quietly spying on Freedom House to see if she could get a handle on what the medics did. It was informative, but what she learned, transmitted through the crackled hiss of a two-way radio, was also dismaying. There was no uniformity in dispatch or response. Patient assessments—detailed, on-scene evaluations of illness or injury—varied wildly, treatment even more so. The crews themselves openly bickered over the air. Much of this she attributed to the effects of a service left too long without a guiding force, but some of her alarm was due to clashing expectations and experience. Nancy had earned her stripes in the strictly calibrated world of the ICU. The medics were practicing something else entirely, a brand of medicine that descended from hearses and cop cars and had been perfected on battlefields and street corners and in the back of wildly careening Cadillacs. Practical considerations present nowhere else (doctors don't drag their unconscious patients out from behind the toilet) forced strange and bewildering realities on street medicine. She would have to fix what she could and learn to harness the rest.

Getting herself and the crews up to speed would be a gargantuan task. Some of it could be handled in the classroom. She'd have a couple hours every day to teach the medics things they would go out and do that night on the streets. But to actually pull the whole thing off, she'd have to intervene personally and become "maximally obnoxious." To get the job done, Nancy would institute what she privately referred to as an "Orwellian reign of terror."

JOHN'S FIRST INDICATION that everything had changed was Nancy's disembodied voice calling to him from the radio. Apparently she was listening on his dispatch, and the moment he arrived on-scene she butted in, demanding to know, specifically, what they found and how they were responding to it. John reached for his radio but said nothing and into the silence Nancy poured advice, critiques, and criticism. When he did respond, his answers either came too slow or off-key, proof in her mind that a mistake was possible. She prodded him, trying to find out what questions he asked, what he did for the patient, and what else he might've missed. It was like someone peering over his shoulder, watching, correcting, chastising. John hardly knew Nancy's name and would've had a tough time picking her out on the street, but already he was scared of her. From that day on, she haunted his calls.

And the radio was just the start. She instituted weekly debriefings where medics were forced to stand before their peers to have every detail of a call dissected. These were held in a classroom deep inside Presby—white walls and blinding overhead lights, a projector, a scale model of a human skeleton, a couple dozen chairs forming a semi-circle. Nancy, pen in hand, sat to the side. The first time John was interrogated, he stepped tentatively into the middle. He was meticulous with his patients—George had loosened him up but not so much that he stopped assessing every patient, even the obviously drunk, for signs of something besides drunkenness. But still.

So now here he was, standing in front of the entire service, Nancy thumbing through one of his call reports. He wasn't sure which one—you had to be ready for anything. John wasn't big on public speaking, but this was worse. It was public defense. Nancy looked up and began reading the report. She'd chosen a chest pain call that he'd recently run, and at first he was confident, relieved almost, because these he knew backward and forward, but then the questions came. A whole flurry of them. What were the vitals? Why hadn't he triple-checked them? How much oxygen had he given? Why? Was there peripheral edema? Did the neck veins show signs of distention? Sure, he listened to lung sounds, but how about heart tones? *No? Why not?* The other medics, knowing they were next, looked away. But Nancy's eyes bore into him. What did the EKG read? What did that tell him? How did he react? Why? Why? Why?

They stumbled out that first day stunned. Guys quickly found excuses not to return. Attendance dwindled so much that Nancy gave money to those who showed up. Grudgingly, they came back, but the cash incentive made the experience no less terrifying or exhausting. They were becoming paranoid, and that was the whole point. She wanted her voice in their heads on every call. Pushing them. Driving them. Slowly she was excising the mistakes and the bad habits, but they didn't have time for slowly. They didn't have time at all.

So Nancy began riding the ambulance.

A suicide, a premature birth, a heart attack at the Carnegie Museum—any emergency coming in over the red phone, and Nancy leapt at it. The first time she trailed John it was to a stabbing on Bedford involving a guy who'd lost so much blood—it looked like all the blood—that neither of them noticed he had a basilar skull fracture until he said he'd also been hit with a bat. Squatting in the filthy house, little kids running in and out, an old woman outside screaming loud enough to be heard through the broken kitchen window, they stared at each other, lost in the silent communion of people who know they've gotten lucky, and that next time, because there's always a next time, they'd have to be better.

Nancy was not only teaching but learning too, and yet her mission to improve Freedom House was only part of why she was out there. Her life beyond work was marked by loneliness and heartache, by doubt. But on an ambulance she could lose herself—"We are a red light flashing along an empty . . . street," she wrote. As a child, she sat next to the piano when her mother played, yelling in protest any time the music stopped. Now instead of music, it was a siren Nancy needed. The ambulance transformed her into a "town crier," its ribbon of sound loud enough to drown everything else out. Like Safar and John, she found salvation in the saving, in its noise and chaos, and chased it into "the squalor and misery . . . the decay, the violence, the depravity." But even this relief was temporary:

> Today I careened through the streets in an ambulance, searching [for] some sign that would ignite my life with meaning.
>
> I returned home again in darkness.

So she rode more. She rode constantly, to the point of exhaustion, and she passed right by it, to disorientation and beyond.

She put a cot in the bunk room, stopped going home, stopped doing anything but running calls until the outside world (finally, thankfully) became an abstraction. She was interested only in emergencies, like a stabbing at the 2000 block of Elmore Square that sent her racing with paramedics Davis and McDoodle through congested streets to a body floating facedown in its own blood that turned out, on closer inspection, even though there were children gawking over it, not to be a dead body but a woman still very much alive, or at least she was until they touched her, at which point she went into cardiac arrest and wasn't *that* inconvenient, considering the knife that sliced into her chest had also punctured her lungs and severed her aorta so that with each compression air leaked and blood spurted and covered them all in a hot sticky mess, though if she were being honest, that was only part of the problem, second fiddle as it were, to the fact that by then the neighborhood had come out to see, and of course they all knew the woman and with nowhere else to focus their grief and rage started raining rocks down on the medics; that was one type of concern, one call, and another was the time Nancy and Ragin happened on a guy covered in blood and who said his enemies were still out there, so as Ragin brought him into the ambulance, people started screaming—"They're coming" and "They've got guns" and "He's got a hatchet" and "They'll kill him"—and then a group of guys who, in fact, did have guns and a hatchet and were, in fact, planning to kill their patient all at once hopped into the ambulance, at which point everything began moving very fast, the sudden violence underscored by gun shots and screams and a hatchet-on-metal clank that drove Nancy scrambling to the front and Ragin slithering out the side and was interrupted only by the growing sound of police sirens, all of this of course being evidence that the job was dangerous, so much so that Safar pulled her aside one morning to say he—along with every nurse in the city—had heard her over the radio the night before as she chased a wounded psych patient through the dark and into an abandoned haunted house of a building, actions he found unnecessary to the job, not to mention reckless and dangerous, and he urged her to stay safe and out of trouble, in other words off the ambulance and out of the base station, but by then she couldn't because with each passing day she got further from where she'd been, more estranged from her fellow doctors by both proximity and lifestyle, to the point they started to complain that she wasn't doing her share of work in the ICU—preferential treatment, they felt, for having accepted a job they'd all turned down—complaints that made their way to Safar, sparking a barbed back and forth between them (Safar questioning her time management, experience, and maturity; Nancy shooting back that fixing a mess left behind by more experienced and mature doctors took nearly all of her time), and though Safar ultimately professed admiration for her dedication, the whole episode represented yet another split from her colleagues, though not one word of this did she share with anyone at Freedom House, where they had no idea of her troubles, so good was she at compartmentalizing that she betrayed nothing, just kept on running calls, kept teaching, kept helping, doing it all with an intensity that made clear she cared about little aside from their ultimate success and in the process earning, slowly, a grudging respect from even the most entrenched medics, from even Walt Brown, whose explosive laugh erupted with such joy it felt to Nancy like life itself, though of course Walt's laugh couldn't overcome the difficulty of the work and the time it stole, the nights she spent on a cot, the nights she never even made it to the cot, the overall effect of which was to bend reality even further—

Too many cigarettes, too little sleep

A state of strange lucidity

The mind outdistances itself and is forever doubling back to pick up stray thoughts

—her schedule not really a schedule so much as a test of human endurance that left her "at the edge of madness," slogging through weeks that were no longer weeks "but a single enormous day" whose boundaries were shaped not by time but emergencies, by an eight-year-old boy knocked senseless from a baseball to the head at Three Rivers Stadium and a middle-aged man mumbling to himself in a filthy bed, by an old woman gasping for air or the lonely wife crying over her dying husband, by the overdose, the diabetic, the gunshot, the children surrounding their unconscious mother, even by the dead body rotting alone in the basement of the ALCOA building and, of course, the diner with chest pain whose server just kept right on serving ("Yours was the filet of sole, wasn't it?"), on and on they came, these calls—heart attacks and assaults, a man who turned out to have a loaded pistol in his jacket pocket just inches from the electrified paddle she used to shock him—and Nancy kept running them, even going down in a sewer with George and Walt (a cop, smug, said it was the perfect call for Freedom House) to shock a man in ankle-deep water—*stand very clear*—and then getting lost on the way back up, a tiny band of pilgrims bearing a second-chance life, emerging from the darkness to find the snow melting, Nancy shaky and giddy from not having slept, blinking in the sunlight, but how could it be dawn—it was never night.

Which is a long way of saying she worked really hard. And her dedication to the job, to the medics, was so complete it washed away whatever boundaries existed between them. She came to know their job and they hers, and through that understanding they got to know one another as people. Nancy wasn't like Safar's other appointees in ways that went beyond the effort she put into her work. She talked and joked, confided, consoled, listened. She ate with them, even the fish sandwiches George got from his favorite restaurant—"place is legit," he assured her—which were so big and greasy everybody joked that someone had gone and killed Shamu.

Since coming to Pittsburgh Nancy had been looking for warmth and friendship, for a purpose, and now, at last, down in the base station and surrounded by the smiling faces of people with whom she'd risked her life, she'd found it.

CHAPTER THIRTY-ONE

The previous year had been a long stretch of ominous weather for Freedom House, and it didn't break, not really, until the spring of '75. It was like a heat wave had settled in and gotten trapped, pushed down by conditions from above, flattening and expanding, growing, until it became a weather system in its own right, sucking in every drop of moisture and leaving only an eerie void that people living on farms in the Midwest or trailers in the southeast refer to as tornado weather. When unsettling stillness finally breaks, it feels, in the moment, sudden. But of course it's been there all along, slowly building.

And it started with the Advanced Life Support (ALS) upgrade class. The class was Safar's idea, his design, though it most definitely wasn't his anymore. It belonged to Nancy now, and the first thing she did was tinker with it—slightly expanding some areas, blowing others out entirely. It'd become about more than education. Now it was about survival, about making Freedom House indispensable, about letting everyone everywhere know they were as good as it got, certainly too good to bury alive. What started out as ambitious in that classically Safar way only got more so in Nancy's hands.

Every day, from eight in the morning until two in the afternoon, medics sat in a classroom in Presby's Scaife Hall, a big concrete sarcophagus of a building, sharpening their knowledge to a fine point. The class was supposed to put a cap on everything they'd been doing, but to get there, Nancy brought them back to basics. She started with a review of anatomy and physiology—this is a heart, here's the aorta—before beelining to what can go wrong (aortic aneurism) and what signs a patient might complain of (lower back pain), finally circling the wagons around what findings to expect on physical examination (unequal pulses). Nancy's teaching style was all about building blocks, foundations, a walk-before-you-run approach that was frustrating for guys who'd been practicing medicine in the streets for seven years.

They pushed back, particularly on Nancy's insistence that they learn the exact wording and cadence doctors use when giving a patient report at the hospital. John in particular didn't understand why they had to know this—half the time doctors laughed or just walked off while he was talking, and if they didn't want to listen, then why bother saying it? This, to Nancy, was exactly the point. She knew how it felt to be overlooked and talked down to. People still referred to her as a "pixie" or "pert" or "a little woman with a big job." The problem might've been with the doctors, but the fix would have to come from the medics themselves.

"If you don't learn to speak like they do," she said, "they'll never stop laughing."

So John kept working, they all did, and Nancy rewarded their patience with access. Every day after class she led them places they weren't supposed to be. All over the hospital, on every floor, through any door. She'd pressure Safar into pressuring someone else into giving them access to whatever forbidden zone she wanted to enter, and if that failed, she'd simply barge right in. They didn't exactly break in, but they weren't always invited either. Nancy just took them.

The dog lab, off-limits to everyone but medical students, was one of those places. Nancy snuck them in one day, quietly divided them by twos, and then gave each pair a live dog. John was an animal lover, but there didn't seem to be any way to get out of this, so he sedated his dog and, while it was unconscious, intubated it. He was marveling at how similar a dog's anatomy was to that of a human when he realized his dog's heart had stopped beating. John immediately started CPR—a use of the technique probably Safar himself never anticipated—and, to his relief, revived his dog.

Day after day they stormed through doors marked "Authorized Personnel Only," heads turning in surprise at the sight of this young white woman and her entourage of Black men. To walk into the Critical Care Unit as if he belonged, to pick up a chart and take vitals, to check ventilator settings and med doses, question nurses, question doctors, to John it was the greatest feeling on earth. He felt ten feet tall. Not bulletproof maybe but something close to it. He came to revere Nancy and would follow her anywhere, believing that anything he needed to succeed she would make happen.

ONE DAY JOHN walked into class, and Safar was there, waiting for him. Really, he didn't know Safar at all. Certainly they'd never spoken. He'd seen the guy and heard everyone else speaking about him in the sort of hushed tones of people who respect but also, and even more so, fear the man they work for. To John, Safar was a suggestion, a whispered name—Peter—as in "Peter thinks," "Peter said," "Peter expects," "Don't make Peter come down here." But now Peter was here. And he'd come for John.

Safar led him to the OR, which John, still uncomfortable around doctors, entered as quietly and unobtrusively as possible after scrubbing in. In front of him was the surgical gurney, and on it lay a patient as ready for surgery as someone could get. Flat on his back, undressed, shaved, and sedated. The surgeon was there, and so was the OR tech. Seated at the head was an anesthesiologist. Beyond them, watching from the amphitheater, was a handful of medical students. John pressed his back to the wall. Everyone surrounding the patient was masked, gowned, and gloved, the whole area sterile. Next to the patient sat an endotracheal tube made of stiff red rubber and a laryngoscope, both within easy reach of the anesthesiologist, who was clearly about to intubate the patient. John was excited. Safar had brought him all the way here just to witness it.

The doctors continued their preparations, and at the last possible moment, Safar told the anesthesiologist to stand up and John to sit down. John froze. He gasped. Fear shot through him—hot at first, then cold as the adrenaline dump hit his bloodstream. Scared as he was, he had no choice. Either do this or be sent home and made to look a fool. So he stepped forward.

A small black stool waited for him at the head of the patient, but when John sat down, it was too low. The anesthesiologist must've been taller, a lot taller, and needed less clearance because, seated, John could hardly see. His mind went blank. Everything he'd learned in Nancy's lectures and the textbooks, all that practice on mannikins, the illicit time spent in the dog lab at Scaife Hall, gone. All of it. *Poof.* He needed to adjust the stool, but there was no time for that. He had a patient not breathing, a surgeon ready for surgery, an amphitheater full of students watching, and, at the center of it all, Safar keeping time. He'd have to make do.

Deep breath, here we go.

The rules were the same as they'd been back in '67, the last time Freedom House medics had tried to pull this off—thirty seconds to successfully place the tube and confirm its position, or else Safar yells time and they'd yank John from his seat. Craning his neck to see, John tilted the patient's head back to open the airway and then blindly reached with his right hand for the laryngoscope. He shifted the tool to his left hand, felt the cold of the metal in his palm, slipped the blade into the patient's mouth, then lifted.

Viewed upside-down, an airway is disorienting. The soft tissue comprising the lower half of the mouth—the lips, the cheeks, tonsils, that giant flopping tongue—all dangle down from a jaw whose organizing musculature has been sent to lunch by the sedative. Like a second grade class whose teacher has left the room, the mouth at this point devolves into chaos. Everything hangs loose and rolls around and must be scooped up and lifted out of the way before you can even peek inside. And even then the task looks far from simple because the pathway to the lungs, which John was anxiously and desperately trying to find, lies directly atop another pathway—the esophagus, leading to the stomach—which isn't just larger but also has yet another loose flap that obscures the target. This flap must also be lifted, but it's awfully far back, and it moves and can be difficult to pin down. Most people, on their first or second or fifth try, thread the wrong opening and end up in the stomach.

John's heart was beating so fast by now the blood was pumping in his ears, and maybe Safar was counting down the seconds, but John couldn't hear it. He could see, though. Just enough. And what he saw when he lifted the blade was the almond-shaped opening of his patient's trachea. Bingo. Now *freeze. Don't blink, don't breathe, don't anything.* He wanted to celebrate or yell, but this wasn't exactly the place for that, and anyway, he was still more scared he'd lose the thing. Ever so slowly, eyes locked on the trachea, he reached for the tube and gently slid it into the patient's mouth, past the tongue, into the throat, and, finally, through the opening and down the airway itself. He was somewhere else now, his muscles moving independently of his mind. The laryngoscope came out; he secured the tube, connected it to the ventilator, and gave one quick puff. The anesthesiologist listened to the sound of air going in, checking to see if the ventilations caused the liquid *gurgle* of air filling the stomach or the steely *swish* of air flowing into the lungs. John waited; Safar waited; everyone waited. Then, with a nod, he said, "Yup, all good," and it was. It was all good. John had successfully placed the tube.

Safar was elated. It'd been a long battle, a personal one, weighted with responsibility, seasoned by failure, but at last they'd gotten there.

The Freedom House medics were intubating. Less than a year after nearly walking away from the cause he had devoted over a decade of his life to, the medics were once again on the crest of the wave. John, the final step of his ALS upgrade complete, walked out of the OR shaken and trembling but smiling from one ear to the other.

CHAPTER THIRTY-TWO

By spring 1975 glimmers of progress were everywhere. In March, Nancy was asked to address the American College of Emergency Physicians at a joint conference held with the Emergency Department Nurses Association. She brought Walt Brown, who demonstrated the sort of advanced life support and airway techniques the medics were learning and putting into practice. Walt was not a common sight among the attendees—big and bearded, with that overcharged personality—but they loved him so much they asked him to come back the next year and do it again. The following month, Freedom House was dispatched to five cardiac arrests and notched a save in every one of them, a remarkable statistic for that or any other time. This did not go unnoticed. Medical directors from services just then getting started made the pilgrimage to Pittsburgh to see what all the fuss was about.

The physician in charge of a paramedic corps based out of Wisconsin's Waukesha Memorial Hospital was so inspired and energized by the two days he spent with Freedom House that he wrote Nancy asking for protocols, histories, or documents of any sort that "would be descriptive of your program or helpful at this point in ours." He was smitten—how could he not be? Everyone else was. Nancy sensed the gathering momentum and wanted to capitalize on the excitement; she decided—on a whim, without consulting anyone else—to put on a massive and very public display of all Freedom House could do. The world needed to know what was happening in the Hill, and the perfect megaphone to amplify their voice was just around the corner and headed their way.

Each May, Pittsburgh played host to an international symposium on trauma and critical care medicine: three full days of experts gathered to discuss innovations and trends that drew a distinguished crowd—Pittsburgh, after all, was home to Peter Safar and Jonas Salk, the virologist who cured polio. Nancy reasoned that with doctors from around the world in attendance, the symposium would be the perfect opportunity to demonstrate just how vital EMS was and, more personally, to make clear that Freedom House was a critical public health resource worthy of respect and, for those keeping score, the DOT grant, which was set to be awarded in July.

Her plan, announced in what Nancy called "a moment of impudent enthusiasm," was for Freedom House to stage a mass-casualty disaster drill on May 8, the last day of the conference, as a sort of night cap to the symposium. It was a big swing, and neither Nancy nor anyone else at Freedom House had ever conceived of, planned for, or tried to pull off something like this before. The problems started immediately.

For starters, Nancy spent hours in vain trying to secure permission to stage her disaster—a multicar wreck—at Point State Park. She had even more trouble finding someone to tow wrecked cars to the scene, wherever it would eventually be, and found herself mired in endless negotiations with the police over crowd control. But the biggest problem by far was practice. Nancy drew up a detailed script for the crash, choreographing where to place volunteer patients whose various states of broken ranged from mildly injured to undeniably dead. Each medic had his own role in the dance, a carefully plotted series of moves to pull off this massive simulated rescue. On paper this should've been the easy part, but they were paramedics, not actors. For providers used to real emergencies, to improvisation, memorizing a staged rescue and making it look genuine turned out to be all but impossible.

They assembled once a week to practice, and each week it got worse. Nancy shouted out instructions, her voice cracking as the scene devolved into a Keystone Kops routine with "half a dozen people running in two dozen directions," most of them performing the wrong care on the wrong patient using the wrong equipment. As D-Day steadily approached, Nancy began to think the disaster drill wouldn't be a drill at all. She went to sleep at night fearing she'd screwed the entire organization, knocking them back on their ass just as they were about to pull off their miraculous turnaround.

As May 8 got closer, preparations remained a mess and were driving Nancy to distraction. There weren't enough cigarettes in the world. Whatever skills she possessed, it was time to acknowledge that conducting the symphony of a large-scale mass-casualty drill wasn't among them. She needed someone more ruthless, more visceral, someone whose size and style inspired both fear and fierce loyalty from the troops. Luckily Freedom House had just such a person.

"I'm giving you the job, Walt." Nancy shook loose a cigarette. Lit it, inhaled. "Do what you like. Just get them in shape."

For the next week, Walt Brown gathered the crews every day. She watched as he "threatened, bullied, shouted, cajoled." If guys hadn't mastered their role, he kept them after practice. A few days later he told Nancy not to worry. "Don't worry, doc. Everything's under control." Walt seemed satisfied, but Nancy was still worried. Any loose thread might unwind a seam and open a hole through which a thousand comic disasters would slip. It could happen, probably would. She was certain of it.

So too was she certain that something needed to be done about the cops.

When Nancy arrived, she was told about, and then witnessed firsthand, the issues Freedom House had with the police. There was little she could do about the nasty things that were said or the contempt with which the medics were sometimes treated—changing hearts was not so simple as restarting them. As they had from the very beginning, cops were still arriving on-scene and stealing patients or not even bothering to dispatch Freedom House at all, even on critical calls. But this she could fix. At least she thought she could. She spoke to the cops, who nodded but didn't change. She spoke to the dispatchers, who gave her assurances but nothing else.

So she tracked down the police superintendent.

In their meeting, Colville was polite but uncomprehending. He himself had spent years on a police wagon, earlier in his career, and saw nothing wrong with how his officers handled medical emergencies. Colville told Dr. Caroline that he couldn't remember a single occasion in which a patient had died from the police providing bad care, a curious oversight in recollection, given the David Lawrence Death Debacle of 1966, but then memories can be like that. Besides, Colville worried any lingering on scene would hurt the image of police as speedy deliverers of care. What patients wanted, he said, what he himself would want, was to be treated by doctors. In a hospital. Not by medics in the street.

Insomuch as there can be a last straw, the Brady Street Bridge was it. Early one morning a Freedom House crew stationed at Mercy Hospital was dispatched to a man who'd fallen forty feet from the bridge—built in 1896, spanning the Monongahela River—and landed facedown on the concrete below. The crew screeched up to find their patient, miraculously, conscious but bleeding heavily from the nose and ear, with a large laceration above his eye. He had severe pain in his back and all four limbs. The list of probable injuries from such a fall was daunting. Facial fracture, skull fracture, brain injury. Hemorrhage of the kidneys, spleen, or liver. Traumatic aneurism, broken femur, crushed pelvis. That's only the start of it. His were the sort of potential problems that required surgery, and what he needed most was a quick ride to the hospital.

But there was one problem the medics could address, and that was the very real possibility of a spinal fracture. This is what they were attending to when, in a scene far too similar to John's dustup with the police over the driver of the VW Beetle, the cops arrived, and immediately the arguing started.

The cops said the man was too injured to leave just lying there and weren't hearing it when the medics explained they weren't leaving him there but packaging him for a safe transport. The cops stepped forward, grabbed hold of the man's belt and hoisted him up. There was a gasp from the Freedom House medics; then the cops swung him onto their canvas stretcher. He was transferred, facedown and alone, in the back of the police wagon to Presby. The medics followed. They arrived just behind the cops and walked into the ER carrying their backboard and immobilization gear. They helped the doctors get the patient onto a gurney and stayed to treat him there in the ER, working alongside the doctors and nurses to start IVs and give fluid. They helped obtain the X-rays that showed the man had broken both wrists, his jaw, pelvis, ribs, and left scapula, and that his mediastinum (the area between the lungs) was widened, which, among other serious problems, can tear the major blood vessels of the heart. X-rays also showed, as the medics had feared, that in falling forty feet onto concrete he'd fractured his cervical spine.

The mood in the base station was frustration. It was anger. Humiliation. It was the sense that even as scrutiny over their actions was more intense than ever, they were too often prevented from acting. The low-pressure system that had been building, filling the air with a sense of anxious anticipation, had finally sucked the last drops of moisture from the atmosphere. And then, at last, it broke.

It happened fast. One day Nancy blew through the door, stalked right over to the dispatch desk, and just as John was walking in, she slammed down a police scanner.

CHAPTER THIRTY-THREE

Four bald tires rolling madly. Speeding around a corner, the ambulance's back end wildly fishtailing. It lurched, wailed, the sound and fury of rescue on its way. The front tire splashed into a pothole, slamming into the divot's front lip with a *thud* that sent a jarring shudder through the van. Nancy's teeth rattled. She was up in the passenger seat. Bill Raynovich drove, one foot pressing the accelerator more or less all the way down. Not even a minute before, a voice had arisen from the scanner announcing an overdose at Elmore Square. They hurried out to the ambulance, hopped in, and were on their way before they realized Raynovich's partner, Dave Rayzer, hadn't followed them out.

No time to wait. They were racing the cops to the scene of a call that by all rights should've been theirs to begin with, a call they knew about only because they heard it go out over the police scanner they weren't supposed to have. The cops, once again, were sending their own units to a critical patient and cutting Freedom House out entirely.

As they rounded another corner, there was a small crash in the back and then a mad scramble. They turned to see Rayzer, shirtless, poking his head up. He'd been sleeping in the back and rolled off the bench. He was up now, confused—"Where we going?" Nancy explained that they had a call, or rather that the police had a call, an OD, and they were trying to steal what was rightfully theirs. Trying but failing. By the time they pulled in, the police were already pulling out.

Nancy flipped off the sirens, and they rolled right by. They lost this one. But there'd be more.

THE DAY NANCY stormed in with the scanner, John didn't even know what it was at first. But then this strange black box with the blinking red lights did something remarkable: with a burst of static from its speaker, the scanner began broadcasting a voice. And not just any voice but a *white* voice. The guy was radioing back not from the scene of a medical emergency but from a crime scene, and John suddenly realized what he was looking at. Somehow Nancy had gotten her hands on this thing, and now it was broadcasting radio traffic from the Pittsburgh police directly into Freedom House headquarters. For years they'd been playing (and losing) an impossible game against the same unbeatable team, and now, with the clock winding down, they'd snuck into the huddle to steal their plays. It was excitement and mischief, and John, thrilled, stood frozen in place.

In short order, the scanner became the focal point of life in the Freedom House base station. They listened to its chatter day and night, waiting for the police wagons to be dispatched on a call, and out they'd go. They were overstepping their boundaries, they knew that, but they were bolder now, and anyway what choice did they have? The alternative was to leave the Hill's most critical patients, those who most needed expert care, in the hands of people determined not to deliver any care at all. That was no kind of choice.

And so the great police races were on.

After the near miss at Elmore Square there was another, a call for a man cut up in a street fight at Fifth and Bouquet. They were out the door quicker this time and drove faster too. Maybe it was that with more police wagons on the street the cops stood a better chance of having a unit close by, and so once again the police beat them. When they screeched up, the guy was already on the cot. His collar bone looked broken, his face bleeding badly. As Nancy hopped out, she could hear him choking on his own blood. The exchange that followed was typical—"You guys need help?" "Nope, we're only two minutes from the hospital." She rolled her eyes. Another two minutes and probably the guy would be dead already.

She needed to intervene but wasn't sure how until the patient's girlfriend, crying, hysterical, jumped onto the cot and threw everything into chaos. Just the opening Nancy was looking for. She elbowed her way into the back of the wagon and manually cleared his airway—if nothing else, at least he was no longer drowning. If the cops were surprised or annoyed, they hardly showed it, just shook their heads and slammed the door, left Nancy in the back of the police wagon and smiling from the window as they drove away.

This wasn't exactly what she'd hoped for, but then it wasn't entirely a loss, either. They were getting closer, firing for range. Winning was a matter of speed and will. Freedom House had the will to win; they knew that. So it would all come down to speed.

AFTER A SERIES of near misses, they were poised and ready to run the instant a call dropped, sprinting out the door and hopping into the ambulance—"Keep the engines running"—and roaring off. It gave the base station an extra jolt of excitement. On any given day, laughter filled the room, where Nancy sat reclined in a chair, hair down, feet kicked up on a desk. Her eyes shining the way they did whenever Walt was on a tear. Whatever funk she sank into, Walt could always pull her out. The base station in general could pull her out. It was loud in there. All the laughing and yelling, the talking, shit-talking, the *yeah, but for real* talking—this is what sustained her. Then a crackle would come from the police scanner, and everyone fell silent to listen.

One night, about three thirty a.m., a call rose from the scanner for a shooting in progress on Burrows. Nancy was on the way before the meaning of the words *shooting in progress* fully set in. Two minutes later she was on the scene, not a cop in sight. There was elation in the ambulance—*We did it! We got here first!*—but only for a second, and then after that came the shooting. A loud crack from the darkness. A pop from somewhere else. Another crack. The whining *twang* as a bullet ricocheted off the ambulance. They hit the floor, panting, too scared to do anything but giggle. In the end, the only thing shot that night was the ambulance, and they left with nothing but a hollow victory.

But more and more they started winning now. They tried to keep it cordial, casual. Nancy and John were packaging a patient for transport when the cops walked up wondering what a Freedom House ambulance was doing there, since they hadn't called for one. Nancy would stand up, friendly smile on her face, a hand shielding her eyes from the sun. "Happened to be in the neighborhood." A shrug like it was all accidental, like the cops couldn't smell the chemical stink of their melted brakes still cooking from the mad dash to get here. "Figured we'd help." Other times they were already leaving by the time the cops showed up. There's John pulling away with his patient as the cops are speeding in. He'd shoot up a big happy wave like "nothing to see here," the cops so confused—*Did he just . . . ?*—that all they could do was wave back.

Late one afternoon the scanner coughed up the particulars of a medical emergency, a call that should've immediately lit up the red phone but didn't because yet again the cops were keeping it for themselves. A man having a stroke at Point Park College. No, check that, a woman, and she was just a few blocks from the Mon Wharf. John, George, and Nancy all piled in, a clown car without power steering, and they were gone. They raced over and found nothing but the cops, who were as confused to see them as they were glad to be there. The moment didn't last long. The cops pulled a hard U-turn and headed for the Hilton. John spun the wheel and followed along. Again they found nothing. The police peeled off, still on the hunt, and as the paramedics discussed what to do next—Nancy poking her head up between them from the back—someone ran over yelling that the patient (a man it turned out) wasn't at the college or the Hilton but up on the bridge. And he was having a heart attack.

John stomped on the gas and spun the wheel with all his might, shoulders on fire, and hit the entrance for the Fort Duquesne Bridge at sixty miles an hour. The engine was screaming, whip antenna swinging like a lasso, as they crossed the river. But the bridge was a double-decker, and their patient, surrounded by a crowd, was on the lower span. So they crossed lanes, got off the bridge, wound their way around to the other on-ramp, and hauled ass to the scene.

The door let out a throaty creak as it swung open. John's feet hit the pavement just as the cops pulled up behind them. Everybody was out at once. John, George, Nancy, two police officers, the bystanders, the patient, passing cars—the whole world. And in that moment the challenge of taking on the cops moved to a new phase. It would be a foot race. John dashed across the bridge and scattered the crowd, only to come to a sudden screeching halt. Everyone else piled in behind, more or less bumping into each other as they froze. Between them and their patient, lying on a pedestrian walkway, was a twelve-foot-high fence topped with razor wire. John stood there, sizing up this latest obstacle, hip to hip with the cops in his white Freedom House tunic, George looking over his shoulder. Nothing to do but do it. John started climbing. Not to be outdone, one of the cops laced his fingers through the chain-link and started up behind him. The fence swayed and bowed beneath the full weight of two grown men. John wobbled, tightened his grip. George clucked—he knew his partner, tireless, devoted to the cause; he could've told you this was going to happen.

John hit the barbed wire. It ripped his jacket and carved shallow ribbons down his forearms. Snared, bleeding, crouched atop the fence, looking down at the churning swirl of the river, he hesitated. The decking of the bridge was fifty feet above the Allegheny River, and he was stuck in a fence twelve feet above that. The wind attacked from all directions, and the fence buckled as the cop struggled below him.

It wouldn't take much for him to slip and topple backward. He could jump wrong and get hurt or jump too far and hit nothing but air. He could've gone back down. Probably he should've.

Instead, he jumped. Landed with a thud, rolled, got up in a crouch and checked to see that he wasn't hurt, then got to work. The patient wasn't breathing, didn't have a pulse, and John began CPR. The cop came tumbling after him. They were eye to eye now, John and this cop, staring at each other over the lifeless body of their patient. It was a tense moment between two men who existed on opposite sides of a seemingly unbridgeable divide. But there was a life to save, and he needed to get on with his assessment, so John showed the cop how to do compressions, and without another word they got to work. George started tossing everything over the fence. Cardiac monitor, oxygen, drug kit. Eventually he came over himself. The cop continued chest compressions, while John and George handled everything else. Shocks and IVs, drugs, ventilations.

How to get him off the bridge would be another magic trick altogether, but ultimately they agreed to carry him down the stairs and meet the ambulance on the frontage road. Nancy raced off in search of a way down, followed by the police wagon. There were a million stairs on the way down, and John and this cop, strange bedfellows, stopped every few steps for compressions. When they finally reached the ground level, the wagon was there but not Nancy—somehow she'd gotten turned around and disappeared—and instead of transporting the patient in the ambulance, they wound up in the wagon. The doors slammed, and John found himself in the belly of the beast.

Surely one of the most surreal moments of his career, but John didn't have time to think about it. Didn't have room to think. In a few moments, they were backing in to the hospital entrance, and then it was the crush of doctors and nurses, the chaotic hand-off of a critically ill patient. Shouts and alarm bells. Calls for orders, for compressions, for time. All of them—John, Nancy, George, and the cops—faded to the back as the hospital staff took over. The silence is always eerie after so much desperate commotion. They washed their hands together in the same big sink. John was exhausted and sweaty, but the cop next to him was still giddy with excitement. As the cop walked off, he turned and waved—a huge smile—said, "We've got to work together more often!"

What is the face of victory? If you had asked John at that exact moment, he would've said it looks something like surprise.

CHAPTER THIRTY-FOUR

On the morning of the disaster drill, it was warm and clear. By noon temperatures reached the upper 70s. A light wind blew along Commonwealth Place, as a hundred people, spread across an entire block, gaped at a collage of wrecked vehicles and critically injured patients. It was quiet enough to hear the soft scuffle of feet, the odd cough. Most were medical professionals in town for the symposium, but there were also, sprinkled among the doctors, startled locals who'd happened upon something strange and extraordinary and wanted to see what it was.

After protracted negotiations with the police for crowd control and with a salvage yard for cars, Nancy had managed to secure a site outside the Hilton. After weeks of worry and work, it was about to start. Maybe Nancy should've felt relief as she squeezed through the crowd to nod at Sol Edelstein, who stood at a podium across the street. The work was done, nothing left for her to do now but sit back and watch. Relief was most definitely not what she felt. She felt terror; she felt dread, anxiety, regret. She felt helpless in the face of certain disaster—real disaster. As Edelstein glanced down at the script she'd written up and begged him to read, her mind whirled and tumbled—she hadn't prepared the medics enough; she had messed up; they'd mess up; this whole thing was a mistake; she had to stop it; she couldn't stop it; it was starting. Here we go.

Feedback squealed through the speakers. Shielding their eyes from the midday sun, the spectators, drowsy, uncertain, craned their necks toward Edelstein. He leaned into the mic and began reading, first walking the crowd through the wreckage, then pointing out the victims and their various injuries—where and how they were broken, who was dead and who soon would be. Of those still alive, fourteen could be saved, he said, but only if someone arrived quickly to save them.

"This is a multi-casualty disaster. Moments ago, these fourteen people were alive and well . . . Now they are casualties. Whether they will live or die depends on the care they receive in the next few minutes."

The distant howl of the first siren broke the noon lull.

"If this happens in your town, would your community be able to respond?" Edelstein asked. "Let us observe what would ensue if this emergency occurred in a city with a fully organized emergency medical system."

The crowd listened as the ambulance drew closer, heard but unseen, nothing but a slow growing wail. Then it rounded the corner. An orange and white blur, chrome and steel glinting in the sun. It screeched to a halt. A second followed. Then a third. They just kept coming.

John threw his truck into park and hit the street running. From the corner of his eye, he could see the crowd riveted to the sidewalk, here to witness what he could do and had done, a thousand times, what he'd do for them if the need arose. Nancy's stomach was in knots, but John loved the attention. He was the kid who'd arrived in town without a change of clothes, who'd been doubted and denied, who clawed his way up—he was still clawing—and now he ran into the action, smiling, eyes on the crowd and thinking, *Yeah, I'm gonna show you what I can do.*

He reached the first victim and dropped to his knees.

All around him it was the same. One by one the medics hit their mark. The crowd didn't speak, didn't move. Patients were assessed and triaged, separated into distinct categories—critical, injured, and walking wounded. The dead were left where they fell. Top priority went to life threats like hemorrhages (tourniquet) and blocked airways (reposition, ventilation). Once stabilized, these patients were quickly rushed off. The critical were then treated with traction splints, spinal immobilization, oxygen, and bandages before being whisked away in the next wave. The stable were treated and released right there on the street.

WHEN THE LAST ambulance pulled away, Nancy looked down at her watch. Freedom House had been dispatched and arrived at the scene of a massive, multipatient accident, had assessed the scene, requested more units, conducted triage, and treated and transported over a dozen patients—all in a hair over twenty minutes. To John, it was no big deal. All in a day's work. The audience had a far different reaction. Hardly anyone present that day had seen an ambulance in action, and most lived or worked in areas where their call for help would reach nothing but a mortician in a hearse.

Laypeople who had no idea such a system existed were amazed by the speed, skill, and organization on display. For doctors, who understood precisely what they were seeing, it was a revelation. They saw what came through the doors of their hospitals each day, and it didn't remotely resemble what they'd seen here today. Hell, they themselves had received only sparse emergency training, and none of it touched on handling life threats in the street. They peppered Nancy with questions and heaped praise on the medics. In the weeks that followed, experts who'd seen them in action and attended their lectures agreed that Freedom House represented "the most skilled and sophisticated [paramedics] in the nation."

Nancy's gamble had paid off. In fact, all their efforts that spring were paying off. In only a few weeks' time, Freedom House would be chosen by the DOT to serve as the model for the standardized EMS training program. The curriculum she and Safar had developed would now serve as the model for paramedic training, effectively making Freedom House the model for generations of paramedics in America, and by proxy the world. In addition, using her time and experience in the Hill as a guide, Nancy would spend the next year immortalizing their work in a textbook that would be used for decades to train EMS students. This service, which had started with a couple dozen conscripts and exceeded all expectations to save lives and open minds in a city that gave them in return nothing but trouble, had become the national standard.

But that was still to come. The day of the disaster drill, when it was finally over, wreckers hauled away the cars, and cops reopened the road. The crowd slowly drifted away. But Nancy stayed behind. She sat on the curb by herself and smoked a cigarette, frazzled, victorious.

IF FREEDOM HOUSE was on the verge of arriving at something greater, so too was John Moon. One afternoon he was dispatched to a call over on Forbes Avenue. The family was there when he and George arrived and guided them into a back bedroom, where an elderly man lay on the floor, motionless except for the heaving of a ragged breath.

As he knelt next to the patient and peppered the family with questions about medical history and medications and what time this started, it became clear his patient was fading fast. The man had congestive heart failure—a heart damaged by time or injury or congenitally bad luck that allows fluid to build up in the limbs, the stomach, and (most ominously) in the lungs. John found fluid in his hands and feet, as well as a wet gurgle when he breathed. His blood pressure was up, heart rate too. His breathing was labored and loud, but at least he was still breathing. Could've been worse, but then *could be worse* is hardly reassuring.

John decided it'd be best to hurry the patient to the hospital, but he was also aware that Nancy was out there somewhere listening.

Waiting. He grabbed his radio and raised her. She answered right away. He gave her a rundown of the patient, expecting her to ask what hospital he was headed to, but instead she came over the air and in a flat tone said, "Go ahead and intubate the patient."

John, radio in hand, patient flopped on the floor where he knelt, shot a look at George like, *Did she really just say that?*

Yes, they'd been through the training, but no one told him that meant he was going to do it for real out on the street. Maybe he was the first, he didn't know, but he was sure there hadn't been many field intubations at Freedom House. Either way, he wasn't ready to do it. Not yet, not here on this man who was still breathing, albeit not well, and who, now that he stopped to think about it, was unconscious and flat on his back and clearly unable to protect his airway and who probably needed *some* intervention from *someone* but (again) from John? Now? Here? He swallowed, then keyed up the radio, opening the airwaves with a crackled burst of static but didn't say anything. His hands were trembling so much he wasn't sure he could hold the tube. If he tried to intubate this guy and messed up, there'd be no one to help him, and the likelihood of a mistake, here, now, felt huge. In fact, now that he was thinking about it, how much had he really learned from intubating dogs or mannequins or even from that time in the OR? Safar had been there too, hadn't he, reducing the possibility of doing any harm to virtually zero? But not this time. This was the real thing. He leaned his mouth toward the radio.

"Um . . . you kinda broke up."

This wasn't true. Not even a little. He heard it; George heard it. The patient, obtunded and gurgling, probably heard it. John waited for Nancy to come back over the air, and when she did, her voice was quiet and uninflected as if she knew perfectly well that he'd heard her and what he needed wasn't clarification but a nudge.

"I want you to go ahead and intubate this patient," she repeated.

And so he did.

What followed was a mad rush. A scramble to do a thousand things, not sequentially as intended, but all on top of each other in a big messy jumble. Who knows who was having more trouble breathing at this point, John or his patient. He reached for his jump bag and dumped its contents—ten million little things that would all have to be picked up and put away before they could leave. Now that he'd been told to intubate the patient, John convinced himself the man was set to die any second (he wasn't), so he started barking orders at George. *Get me this, get me that—get me another; I just broke this one.* George took it in stride—he understood what was going on. John was moving so fast that when he tried to lubricate the breathing tube, he accidentally lubed his hands, lubed everything, covered it all with a greasy covering of Vaseline. Everything he needed was now slippery.

George put the laryngoscope in John's hand, practically guiding him toward the patient's mouth. John leaned forward, looked in, slipped the tube past the teeth and then on down into an opening at the back. But this wasn't an OR or even a lab; it was an old house in the Hill, and the lights were crap, and where the tube went exactly, well, who could tell? Not John. He was still staring into the darkness of the patient's mouth when George handed him the bag valve mask. John connected it to the tube, fingers slick and covered with carpet lint, and gave the ventilator a quick puff.

The chest rose. *Thank God, thank George, thank this man for having cooperative anatomy.* John connected him to oxygen, started an IV, loaded the guy onto the stretcher, and was on his way out the door. He had only one thought in mind and that was *Let's get the hell outta here before something goes wrong and I kill this man.*

On another day, that might've been the end of the story, but on this day, the day John got his first field intubation—possibly even Freedom House's first field intubation—there was yet another turn.

John didn't hear what the family said as they left or how George responded—his adrenaline was pumping too hard, heart hammering away in his chest. Even on the ride to the hospital he wasn't paying attention to where they were going, just that the lectures and the mannequins, the OR, Nancy's constant badgering, it'd all paid off. Not only because he had managed to intubate the patient but because now that the tube was in and needed to be monitored, he realized he could do it—was doing it—and that he was comfortable and in command. He relaxed.

But eventually they pulled up at the hospital and burst through the doors, and when they did, he realized the patient's family hadn't chosen Presby or Mercy but Montefiore. The hospital where it all started, the exact place that five years before he'd seen a paramedic for the first time, the place where he'd been an orderly, the lowest man in the room, witness to the magic happening around him. Now he was back, wearing the crisp whites of a Freedom House medic, arriving with a critical patient being supported by an advanced intervention that he himself had performed. And it was that intervention—amid his moment of fear and adrenaline and accomplishment—where suddenly and pointedly all the attention went.

"What is this?"

John looked up, confused. His eyes darted across the shocked faces of assembled staff until they fell on the attending physician—stiff, ramrod straight, rooted to the floor, an accusatory finger pointing at the tube.

"Why is this patient intubated?"

Where a moment before it was chaos and motion, there now was nothing. The doctor stared at John, eyes burning a hole through his chest.

"Who did this?"

John said nothing, and the room filled with a silence stretching all the way back to January, when Nancy first arrived. From day one she'd been battering and badgering, questioning, correcting, pushing, punishing, then pushing some more. All the calls she'd listened in on or rode along with, the classes, the weekly debriefings, the patient reports. It was all so exhausting. Half the time it didn't even make sense.

But all along something was gathering, so slowly he could hardly feel it. It was there each time she opened a door they weren't supposed to enter, a growing sense that they belonged and they were vital, a determination—certainly for John, at least—to channel a lifetime of anger and frustration into the power he'd need to reach the top. And the top wasn't a bit of knowledge or a skill—Nancy knew he could intubate, that it was only a matter of time for that part.

In fact, the top wasn't for the patients at all but for the medics themselves. She was demanding and authoritarian, impossible, encouraging, devoted and insistent, because she knew this moment would come. That after John had intubated that first patient and brought him into the hospital, he'd be questioned and doubted. That they all would. The world was waiting for them to fail. Expected it. They weren't from central casting, didn't look the part and definitely didn't fit in, and so good enough was never going to be enough. They'd have to be better than anyone, all the time, just to be accepted. Pulling that off would take a level of supreme confidence that couldn't be faked.

That's why she opened doors. Not just for the access or the resources, but to reinforce the belief they were as good, better, than anyone else who walked through those doors. It's why she brought in Safar for the intubation test. It was on her urging that Safar arrived that day—and on other days—and plucked John out of class.

At that time, in the mid-'70s, doctors functioned on a privileged plane, held in too high a regard to be questioned. And among doctors, none in Pittsburgh were held in higher esteem than Safar. When Safar had led him into the OR that day, John immediately noticed how everyone stopped what they were doing. How all eyes shot to Safar, as if the person in charge of the people in charge had just arrived. They looked at him with deference, spoke to him with reverence. And this man had made time for *John*. Even the medical students had to watch from their seats in the amphitheater, but John was at the head of the patient, part of the surgical team. Safar's guy. And what did that say about him? Everything. It said maybe he wasn't on the same level as those doctors, but he wasn't too far below them either.

That's what Nancy was doing. Making them feel worthy enough to stand up to whatever came their way. It might've been her job to carry them to the door. But it'd be on them to kick it down. And now John was at the door.

He looked up at the doctor. "I intubated him."

It was all so clear now.

The doctor flashed with anger, squared up with him. "And you are?"

Nancy hadn't been building a foundation. She was constructing a pyramid, and this was the peak.

"My name's John Moon. And I'm a paramedic at Freedom House."

BOOK FIVE

CHAPTER THIRTY-FIVE

Maybe it was all a dream. Some fantastic by-product of a time (the '60s!) when everything was possible. Or a hangover maybe, a flashback or hallucination, something you had to come down from (*with the right kind of eye you could almost see the high-water mark*) because only yesterday it was the spring of 1975 and Freedom House was on a magical run, capped, improbably, in July when they were awarded the DOT contract. Through hard work, this group of young men from the Hill had risen from neglect and near collapse to be chosen, and in that moment it seemed there was no way the city could disown or disband them, not now, not after all this. The mayor would finally have to accept Freedom House for the jewel it was. Perhaps even embrace it.

But maybe John had imagined all that because here it was, a year later, and everything was over. Just as Freedom House was being recognized across the nation and beyond, just as it reached the zenith of its powers, it was cut down right here at home. In the span of just a few months, John lost his white Freedom House jacket, his beard, his rowdy coworkers, Freedom House itself. Standing in its place was an ambulance so brand-new and expensive John was almost afraid to touch it, and on its side, in big letters no one could possibly miss, the words *City of Pittsburgh EMS*. The only constant was John himself, who was stepping down from the back of this new ambulance, making his way to yet another house. They were on a call, chest pain, when he was stopped. The medics he was riding with, the city's guys, white guys, nodded toward the open back doors and said, "Grab the bag." That was his job now. He was to stand there, quietly, not touching patients or directing care, not serving as a paramedic or even an EMT but just *standing there*. They didn't see it coming and almost couldn't believe it once it arrived; that's how fast it happened. But it happened. So now John stood there. Holding the bag.

IF YOU LIFT the needle from the record and drop it back in time to May 1975, when the end really became clear, the first sound you catch is City Councilman Robert Rade Stone, a stalwart critic of Flaherty on the ambulance question, mid-sentence, wondering "how many more lives could've been saved if we had moved faster on this program."

Stone was reacting to Flaherty's announcement, made earlier in the day, that he'd finally decided what Pittsburgh's ambulance service would look like going forward. Not that you didn't see this coming on some level, but it wouldn't look anything like it had. In a way, this announcement had been a long time coming. Nancy and Safar had been staring at City Hall with the sort of wary eye an islander might cast upon a long-dormant volcano that's recently started smoking—they knew something was coming but weren't sure what or when or just how catastrophic it would be. All they could do was prepare. Everything they did that spring—the staged disaster, the DOT contract—was at least partially aimed at an audience of one. And for months Flaherty was silent. After reluctantly agreeing to fund the service through the end of the year, the city had acknowledged the existence of Freedom House only once in 1975, and that was to saddle them with the Inebriate Program—an initiative that made transporting the drunk and unruly off the street and into care facilities the sole responsibility of Freedom House.

So it came as something of a surprise on the first of May when the mayor emerged to announce he'd finally created a plan for Pittsburgh

EMS. In fact, several things about it were surprising. First among them was that it would be well funded. No longer would the city skimp on money or allow federal grants to slip away. A whopping $3 million was allocated to the effort to cover its first thirty months. Clearly, financial concerns that once mattered so much were being pushed aside. So were the doctors and experts who'd spent a decade trying to make street medicine a priority. In a surprise move that perhaps shouldn't have been so surprising, Flaherty chose not to make use of Presby's hard-earned knowledge, and he completely ignored Safar, who was recognized worldwide as an authority on emergency care and had spent the last decade designing, training, and running one of the best ambulance services on the planet. Instead, the mayor partnered with Central Medical Pavilion, a downtown hospital whose physicians were new to EMS.

Then there was the question of who.

The city's five new "super ambulances," $35,000 units inspired (as most then were) by Safar's designs, would be staffed by civilians. This was a stunning turnaround. For years the mayor had insisted ambulance care should be run through the police, but now he was making EMS its own branch of public safety, with a half-million-dollar payroll covered by "federal manpower funds." For Freedom House, this was the rare bit of hope rising from City Hall. If the mayor had stuck to his insistence that only cops could ride ambulances, it would've meant certain death. But he didn't. Through doors that'd long since been slammed in their faces, there now emerged a tiny crack of daylight.

Unfortunately, when they crept close enough to peek through it, what they saw was both peculiar and oddly familiar.

"I NEED, FAIRLY urgently, to get some consistent statement from you." This from Nancy to Safar, just a few weeks after the mayor's announcement. "Our people are under considerable pressure and I need to be able to give them rational advice." The note was handwritten on a piece of Safar's own stationary as if the message was too urgent to send through the normal channels, and instead Nancy barged into his office, found it empty, and scrawled out an SOS before nailing it to his door.

Communiqués of this sort—blunt, despairing—flowed regularly from Nancy to Safar over the summer of 1975. All this pressure and its corresponding need for rational advice stemmed not from the fact that the city had announced its own service but that they'd already begun staffing it. It wasn't even that really: it was who they were and weren't hiring. The advanced life support course Nancy and Safar launched the previous winter was held in cooperation with the Community College of Allegheny County. This not only helped with logistics and accreditation but also opened the class to a wider group of students. These students, mostly white guys from suburban and rural communities, sat through Nancy's lectures alongside John and the others and then did their training rides at Freedom House.

When they came, John did his best to make them feel comfortable, but it quickly became clear they needed more than moral support. They didn't have the experience that the Freedom House medics had. Even the ones who'd worked on an ambulance had done so in places that saw fewer emergencies and ran fewer calls. They hadn't been invited on any of Nancy's field trips through Presby. Safar never tapped one of them to intubate patients in the OR. Pulling up on the scene of an emergency, the students would turn wide-eyed to John and ask, "What do you want me to do?"

John answered their questions and helped them manage life threats and chaotic scenes, did what he thought was the right thing, never once thinking he might be training his replacements. Like everyone else, John figured once the class was over these guys would go back to whatever town they'd come from.

But that's not how it went at all. When the city started hiring, they did what seemed impossible then and seems so painfully inevitable all these years later. They took the newer and inexperienced students, the white guys, first.

Much of the new city program had roots in Freedom House. Glenn Cannon, whom Flaherty tapped as director of his new ambulance service, was one of the white guys who'd gotten his start with Freedom House. So was his deputy. Frustrating as this was to watch, John never once considered leaving. He still believed if the core group held on, they'd be able to save Freedom House. But it was beyond galling that their eagerness to further the cause of medicine was taken advantage of and their ALS class treated like a Trojan horse.

When the announcement from the DOT came in July, the moment that was meant to be their grand triumph, the coup that saved them, Nancy and the rest of Freedom House barely noticed. Despite the role it would play in the long-term legacy of both, for the moment the only thing that mattered was saving their jobs. And it was clear the DOT contract—history-making accomplishment or not—wasn't going to help. "During those years that Freedom House was the proving grounds for national standards, everyone had wanted to be part of the act," Nancy wrote. Now they were gathering to dance on its grave.

EVEN AS THE future of Freedom House's experienced medics was cast into doubt—when pressed about hiring the rest of Freedom House's staff, Cannon expressed indifference—an offer came in for Nancy. After thumbing its nose at Pennsylvania's only collection of experts in running exactly the type of service they were now trying to create, city officials were realizing they'd need *someone* who knew what they were doing. And so Nancy was offered the job of medical director.

She turned to Safar for guidance, writing to tell him that after giving the offer "considerable, uneasy thought," she decided that her "answer must be conditional."

Really there was only one condition, and it was simple: Nancy wanted her people hired. They'd just gone through an exhaustive course and acquired a particularly sophisticated skill set, and it would be "madness" for the medics to find themselves unemployed "while less skilled, less experienced individuals . . . have comfortable jobs aboard the city's MICUs." If Flaherty truly wanted her, he'd have to hire every Freedom House employee who wanted to join. "My first commitment is to Freedom House and its personnel. I have no interest in a city-wide service in which they are not a part."

As Nancy considered her future, Safar encouraged forbearance. He commended her "laudable" efforts on behalf of the staff but worried over the cost of her fierce loyalty and gently insisted the job must "ultimately be more than missionary work." Here perhaps was the greatest disconnect between two doctors who would remain lifelong friends and seemed otherwise to be cut from the same cloth. For Safar it had always been about advancing the medicine, even now. But Nancy, who had more than proven her commitment to that goal, also shared Hallen's vision: the people mattered. By now Safar knew this, and whether he truly believed she'd actually listen to him is questionable. Since arriving in Pittsburgh, Nancy had never yielded so much as an inch to Safar. And even on the issue of her own well-being they couldn't agree. This was more than just rebelliousness. Nancy insisted it was she who'd been saved, that she owed a debt to the people of Freedom House—who had, only quite recently, carried her through the rocky waters of unspeakable tragedy.

CHAPTER THIRTY-SIX

It happened in March 1975. Just a couple months before the victories to come, the conference, John's intubation. Just as the world was finally thawing from a long dark winter, as life was returning to the frozen city, hope inching into Nancy's sleepless nights, it was then that Manny's demons rose up to haunt the frayed edges of her life.

It's possible by this time their relationship had entered a new, terminal phase—there were no more poems or cards, no letters about walking along the Charles River. When she wrote to Manny, she wrote of his drinking, his anger, his depression and suicidal thoughts. How he was cruel with alcohol, cold and distant without it. A typical night at home: two in the morning, smell of wood smoke and music drifting in from some other apartment, Nancy jolted awake by a ringing phone, by Manny threatening to take his own life. You can see how (not) sleeping on a cot was easier.

To those who knew him, including his therapist, he was "maddening," a "likeable" guy who "harbored a wild man inside him." He was full of "flamboyance and rage." He was a hard man to live with, harder still to understand. His wife, back home with their children in Kansas City, felt she never really knew him. She was aware of Nancy and her relationship with Manny but bore no resentment. In her eyes Manny was always "reaching for somebody." If that somebody was Nancy, so be it.

The problem was that not even Nancy could reach him. Not anymore. Manny kept too much locked inside. He was filled with a sadness she tried but failed to penetrate. Her efforts, like those of Manny's wife, of his therapist and colleagues, were in vain. She became increasingly worried about him. She intervened personally; she got others to intervene. Her efforts only drew Manny's wrath, but she held firm. Their conversations took on an Alice in Wonderland quality—he once accused her of trying to ruin his dog's life. Nancy was angry and exhausted, hurt, desperate. She wanted to leave him but couldn't. Finally, in the most horrible of ways, Manny did the leaving for her.

The news, heartbreaking, horrifying, arrived as a shock: Manny ingested ammonia and then repeatedly stabbed himself. He was dead. Nancy flew to Boston. She made arrangements; she contacted family and friends; she asked her mother to guide his children around Boston when they arrived for the funeral. She grieved. And then she returned to Pittsburgh, unable to shake the torturous vision of his death but hoping "one day some defense mechanism will come to my rescue."

She told no one at Freedom House. She ran from the hideous images, the raw brutality of Manny's death, and that running brought her straight into the waiting arms of Freedom House. She buried her grief in work, her loneliness in the mad clamor of the base station. She wrote that this "massive dose of human tragedy" left her "disillusioned with mankind in general" and "on the verge of quitting this program and this city altogether."

> Indeed there was nothing that could've kept me here had I not . . . found myself suddenly among genuine, warm human beings again. Down in that base station I discovered an outpost of honesty, camaraderie . . . generosity of spirit. The Freedom House people kept me alive—or at least kept alive in me some shred of faith. And for that I owe them.

The medics were more than just one part of a quest to make ambulance work succeed, more than employees or coworkers or even friends. She'd met their families, risked her life with them, "praised them, berated them, laughed with them, cried with them." When she needed them, even if they didn't know it, they pulled her back from the abyss. *Will you dive after me if I sink too deep?* The debt she now felt far outweighed any risks to her own career. "There are thirty human beings at stake," she wrote to Safar, "and they count for more than any title the city or university can bestow on me."

She vowed to be the last one out the door, to battle for her people regardless of the cost. "You entrusted me with Freedom House and I will see it through to its conclusion."

CHAPTER THIRTY-SEVEN

Nancy wasn't the only one compartmentalizing. Shoving aside fears and concerns, frustrations, humiliations—any negative thoughts at all—had become a Freedom House family tradition. It's how the medics survived their encounters with the police and with racist patients, with a combative administration in City Hall. It's what allowed them to speed around Pittsburgh in ambulances whose engines might, if the mood struck, catch fire. Quietly shouldering a burden and internalizing all of his fears had become a way of life for John, a survival mechanism—learned in the orphanage—that he leaned on now. Freedom House teetered on the brink of collapse, and it broke his heart, but he never let it show. John took pride in his ability to handle hardship and turmoil, even a total lack of control, without showing so much as a trace of emotion. At the time, he took this as evidence of self-reliance but admits, years later, it must surely have felt to Betty like isolation. His refusal to talk or share, to let anyone else in at all, would eventually tear them apart, but in the summer of 1975 it was what allowed him to keep going.

The end had become a freight train barreling down the tracks, and he now found himself unable to ignore that deep rumble rising up from under his feet. He knew why it was happening, the reason the city had never embraced Freedom House and was now planning to scuttle the service, but that didn't matter now. Just as it didn't matter that the medics had done everything that could've been asked of them and then some. The outcome was the same, and so the question became a simple one: If none of what came before mattered, then did running calls still matter? Did the patients matter? Did he?

"It happened like this once before."

These words, whispered to John one night during a call on Bedford Avenue, seemed to encapsulate the larger moment, dragging the lessons of history out of the past and right into the present. On this particular night, John was crammed into the landing of a narrow staircase. Outside, a crowd had gathered to watch, and with the whole neighborhood wobbling in the red bounce of their emergency lights, the mood was almost festive. But in here it was quiet and dim, colorless. George lay at his feet, having just been knocked backward down the stairs with a big crash, all kinds of shouting, a chorus of *oohs* and *ahs* from the spectators, to land there in a heap.

They had been dispatched to a man who'd become violent, and when they found him—atop these stairs, half-buried in the shadows—George went up, just to see what the problem was, to talk. Years after they'd started working together, John could perform all sorts of medical wonders, but there was still nothing quite so effective as George talking. Once he got up there, the patient let out a karate sound (*hwuaaa . . .*) and followed that with a sharp yell (*hiya!*) and punched George in the face. And so, George tumbling down the stairs. And so, the crowd yelling. And so, a bystander whispering that it happened like this once before.

And the last time it happened? "Put him in Western Psych for thirty days."

Another man squeezed into the landing claiming to be the patient's best friend. "He's a karate expert," the best friend said. "Black belt." This shed some light on the situation, but they still didn't know what to do, so the best friend offered to go up there and talk to the patient himself. George stepped to the side and spread his arms out wide like *go right ahead, best friend*. The best friend went up the stairs and from the bottom they heard it all again—the growl (*hwuaaa . . .*), the cry (*hiya!*), and the crash of the best friend tumbling down the stairs.

John sighed and peered up into the darkness. Squinted at the outline of a figure just barely visible in the shadows, then started up the stairs. Not because he thought he could do something the others couldn't, but simply because it was his turn. The whole thing felt eerily familiar, all this going up just to get knocked back down—Sisyphus in a Pittsburgh housing project—but he went anyway. And sure enough, when he got to the top, here came the growl. *Hwuaaa . . .*

On and on it went.

Maybe none of them were surprised that Freedom House was shutting down. But they were angry. They talked about it—the unfairness, the ugliness, the deceit, the stupidity—every minute of every day. Bill Raynovich simply couldn't understand why the city hadn't just taken it over. "You've got a jewel; the whole world is looking at this. Nancy Caroline's writing the manual. She's got the grant. It's being memorialized in the actual literature at the highest levels. How can they do this?"

John spent hours in Nancy's office trying to make sense of what was happening and what to do next. Maybe he should quit, go back to Montefiore and see if they'd hire him on as an orderly.

"Is that what you're going to do?" she asked. "Throw in the towel?"

John, who had a family at home and obligations to meet, nodded his head. "I mean, I'm in a position where I probably have to go back if we're going to shut down."

Nancy was determined to stay until the end, refused to go quietly, and she urged him to do the same. If the Freedom House personnel stuck together, she hoped, made enough noise, the city would be forced to hire them on. They'd made history here and earned the right to keep working, even if it was in a city uniform. When John balked, Nancy asked him to consider what would happen to the people of the

Hill, their patients, if, when Freedom House closed, the paramedics disappeared too. "You can't give up. People will suffer if you quit." So he stayed.

Over the course of the summer, Nancy managed to persuade most of the medics to stay, arguing the importance of their mission but also promising that at the end, when the city took over, there'd be jobs for them too. Now she needed to deliver. Since the city still showed no particular interest in recruiting the Freedom House medics, Nancy played her one remaining card.

One day in the base station she told John it was time to push back.

"Yeah, but how do you do that?"

"One thing about municipal government," she told him. "It does not like negative publicity."

Way back on the night she was first approached about joining Freedom House, stuffed in among the papers shoved into her hands were dozens of clippings from the very public and heated battles between Safar and Flaherty. They told the story of an ugly standoff, and in the end the mayor blinked first—whether or not it was the one he wanted, Safar got his citywide ambulance service. Now that paramedics at last had Flaherty's stamp of approval, Nancy gambled he'd be "anxious to avoid . . . another 'ambulance controversy' in the press."

She put together a list of demands; if the city met them, she'd accept their offer to become medical director. If they didn't, she had a backup plan: she'd reach out to her contacts in the media, to community groups and activists, and begin spilling inside information about members of the political and medical community, stories about people who'd enriched themselves at the expense of Freedom House, which was in part publicly funded. She told Safar about her intentions, explained that she didn't want to cause him any trouble but saw no other alternative. Safar let her know he considered this move to be "blackmail" but nonetheless offered his blessing. "I will be on your side of the barricades as far as Freedom House EMT's future is concerned," he wrote.

THE MASTHEAD ON official Freedom House Enterprises stationary was unexpectedly flowery, the words *Freedom House* arcing across the top in a font that feels more at home on a college diploma than a letter sent by anyone in the last three hundred years. But it did lend an air of grace and officialdom to the terms of surrender Nancy sent to Flaherty. The organization, she wrote, was willing to give the city two ambulances and all of their equipment, plus her own services, free of charge, during the transition period. In return she asked for the following: that the paramedics be hired by Pittsburgh EMS and allowed to practice immediately at their current certification level without further testing; that any Freedom House employee who hadn't yet completed the ALS upgrade course be allowed to do so (and be paid while doing it); that those in school be given a shift conducive to continuing their education; that the dispatchers be hired on in their current role; and that Freedom House employees be allowed to continue working in the Hill and Oakland to maintain the rapport they'd established with the community. She added one final demand, symbolic, but every bit as important as the others: "the city will arrange for a formal ceremony, with press coverage, to mark the transfer of services from FHE to the city, and to acknowledge the service FHE has rendered the community over the last eight years."

Flaherty accepted Nancy's terms. All of them, that is, except the last. Anyone from Freedom House who chose to join the city's new service was free to do so. But there would be no official recognition of the ground they'd broken or the service they'd been providing since 1968. Freedom House would simply disappear.

CHAPTER THIRTY-EIGHT

The end doesn't always feel like it. People come and go; they slip through the door when you're not looking and never come back. Sometimes there are no goodbyes. But Freedom House had an approximate date of execution (mid-October), and the end, in a strange way, dragged on. Bob Zepfel wrote a letter to Nancy—"you'll always be our Doctor One"—and another to Safar—"though we will be disbanded, I'm sure our achievements will not be forgotten." Fittingly, the goodbye letter to the staff was written by Nancy. Accolades after the fact can feel empty, but it says something that several of the medics kept their letter, through the decades, even as their lives wound off in different directions. They lost touch with each other but never the memories. As they went about their final days, Nancy's words hung in the air.

"All of you have reason to be proud. . . . You have taken a dream and made it real."

Even as the new city ambulances began prowling the streets, the medics showed up to work every day and slipped on their white Freedom House jackets.

"You have profoundly affected thousands of lives: the young and the old, the wealthy and the indigent, the prominent and the anonymous."

They continued to run calls. Ragin and Rayzer. Walt, George, Raynovich, and John.

"It has been a rare privilege to know all of you. How grateful I am for your friendship and how honored by the confidence you have shown in me."

One afternoon, just before the end, a child was hit by a bus in one of those wealthy neighborhoods that Freedom House had been barred from entering. The first cop to arrive on the scene panicked.

"If you take with you into the future the dedication and spirit and pride which you have shown in your work here, you will keep alive all that is meaningful and important about Freedom House."

From their pirated police radio, the medics heard the cop scream over the radio, "There are pieces of his leg all over the street. Send Freedom House!" Nancy and a pair of medics jumped into an ambulance and punched the gas.

"Freedom House should be a symbol to all of you what you can achieve despite enormous odds."

The call was out of their area, and another ambulance was closer, so the dispatcher tried to cancel Freedom House. The cop, a member of the very department that had battled them for years and had stood, in many ways, for every stereotype the medics had worked to dismantle, kept screaming for Freedom House. "We need someone who knows what the hell they're doing!"

"This is the end of a grand adventure, the end of a dream that was born eight years ago."

It was one final victory. The recognition refused them by the politicians but granted by those who'd actually been there on the streets, against them, with them.

"But it need not be an end at all. You have proven yourselves."

CHAPTER THIRTY-NINE

On the night of October 15, 1975, everyone gathered in the glass-walled base station at Presby. Their faces were blank. Expressionless. For once the ambulances outside were quiet, the automatic doors didn't swing open to let in any cold air. Not a word was said. When the digital clock flipped over to 11:59 p.m., everyone turned their eyes to Bob Zepfel, who'd been with Freedom House since the beginning, as he picked up the receiver and dialed the police dispatcher. Behind him the medics, dressed for the last time in their white Freedom House jackets, shifted about. Zepfel gripped the phone.

"This is Mr. Zepfel, manager of Freedom House ambulance service. It is now 11:59 p.m. As agreed with the City of Pittsburgh, we are now going off the air."

Slowly, people began to shuffle out. John stared through the window into the night sky. He wondered what it had meant, what it would all become. Whether anyone would remember them. Eventually he, too, left. They all did, except Raynovich, the token hire no one had expected to last a week, let alone to the bitter end. He stayed and kept an eye on their stuff until Mitch Brown showed up in the morning. Not because he had to, just because it felt right. He wanted to honor the job, to follow through. To close the doors.

A COUPLE WEEKS later—after Freedom House but before they started with the city—someone threw a party, and everybody showed up and very quickly what started out as a somber it's-good-to-see-you-what've-you-been-doing type of thing turned into more or less everyone getting drunk and staying all night dancing and laughing and hugging the way you only do around people you've been through too much with and you swear you'll never forget but who, invariably, head off in different directions. Nancy got drunk on Scotch, and when Walt told her that had she come seven years earlier, she might've saved the place, she told him he had it all wrong and that he and everyone else "showed me the way back to something I had lost and did not know how to find." But she felt a lingering bitterness too. "Eight years. The federal standard for ambulance design and equipment. The federal standard for EMT and paramedic training. Eight years. 50,000 runs. How many people, not only in Pittsburgh, but all across the country, owed their lives to the pioneering work done by Freedom House over eight years? I cannot escape the feeling that they were cheated."

Nancy stayed until three in the morning, right about the time it became clear that all the drinks in the world couldn't wash away the heartbreak of the end.

John wondered how many of these people he was hugging and trading war stories with, these people swaying and dancing alongside him, remembering the good and the bad, the unmentionable, how many of them would he ever see again. Wherever they went, whatever became of them after this night was over, John told himself that the world would remember. Had to. They'd done too much for too many, and whatever happened from here nobody could take that away from them.

Right?

CHAPTER FORTY

From the very beginning, the city did what it could to take it all away. All those assurances from the mayor himself that Freedom House staff would be treated fairly once they came over, they turned out to be hollow words. "Over the ensuing months," Nancy later wrote, "all of these promises were broken."

The first hint of things to come happened to Mitch Brown. Cannon offered him a job as second-in-command of the citywide system, a position that would require Mitch, who'd once been Cannon's boss, to swallow his pride. But he accepted because somebody would need to look out for his people and if not him, then who?

The moment Mitch accepted, Cannon called back to say that the job had changed and instead of being second-in-command of the entire organization, the best he could promise was a spot on an ambulance as a crew chief. Take it or leave it.

Mitch left it—would eventually leave the city entirely—and walked away, more wary than ever of what lay ahead. Just a few days later, he addressed an organization of Black professionals and warned that the "warmth" and the "empathy" of the Freedom House days was over. If you called an ambulance for help, he said, "the only way you'll be able to tell them from cops is they won't be carrying guns."

John stood in front of his mirror and slipped on the new uniform he'd been issued. Light blue shirt and dark blue pants. A cop's uniform without the gun, all right. He dressed without ceremony or emotion. There was no pride in these clothes. As he left home and drove to work that first day, he passed over streets that never recovered from the violence of 1968. Burned-out buildings had been bulldozed but never replaced, leaving big swaths of the Hill vacant. Even Centre Avenue, the community's main artery, remained barren, dominated by a large and unruly stretch of mud slowly freezing around a bulldozer—evidence of a grocery store (it'd be the only one) planned but not yet built.

In the remnants of the Hill, John felt the sense of a never-ending loop. What once was theirs had been taken away and divvied up, used by others, and whether it was a neighborhood or an ambulance service, the result was the same, and so was the feeling. *Here we go again.* But John wasn't here to wallow or reminisce or even rebel. He wanted only to be part of the organization, to be accepted as a man and a medic and above all else to serve the community. He was a medical professional, and forget the color of his uniform or the ambulance, the name on the paycheck—some things didn't change. Put him out on the street, and he'd do what he was born to do. He'd save lives.

His first station was in the West End, over a bridge and across the Monongahela River, a white part of town John didn't even know existed. There weren't designated EMS stations, so John's ambulance was posted at a firehouse where it didn't really belong, and rather than being invited in, he and his new partners (both white) had to sit outside in the truck bay with their coats on, huddled up next to a radiator. This shared deprivation did not bring them closer. When John walked in that first night, one of the medics had turned to the other with a look of profound confusion.

"Who's this?"

A sideways glance, quick shrug: "Oh. That's one of the people from Freedom House."

So no "welcome aboard" then. John climbed into the ambulance to see what he was working with and was stopped cold by what he found.

The mayor's super-ambulances were indeed super, every bit of $35,000 worth of new and improved. And equipped? They were equipped with everything you could ask for—in fact they were equipped with everything Freedom House *had been* asking for but never got because it was supposedly too expensive. It was one of those rare moments where everything crystalizes and becomes clear.

John sank into the bench seat and for the first time in years felt entirely alone.

IF HE'D ASKED his former colleagues, they would've told him they all felt the same. Most of Freedom House's staff had come over to work for the city, and they were all going through the same thing. When Raynovich arrived, he looked around and saw the white guys who'd been in Nancy's ALS upgrade class, totally inexperienced medics who joined the city back in the spring and were already its favored sons. He on the other hand, a white medic with five years' experience—plus his time as a marine—was treated like a pariah. On his first day and every day after, for months, he endured an endless parade of nasty looks and snide comments from his new coworkers and even leadership, who he likened to "a goon squad." He was just another employee the city had only begrudgingly taken on, one of *them*, Freedom House, white only on the outside.

The Freedom House medics were told to watch and learn from their new partners, that the city medics were there to mentor them. The idea of being mentored by medics so hopelessly new they didn't yet know how much they didn't know seemed like a joke whose setup was even worse than the punch line because there wasn't any mentoring going on—just a lot of sneering from guys who felt superior because Freedom House was gone and now they were in charge.

Of those first days after the transition John could only say, "I became a second-class citizen."

AT LEAST JOHN was on an ambulance. Not doing the work, maybe, but still around it. The same couldn't be said for the dispatchers, who were assigned to different jobs entirely. Which jobs? Any jobs. Each was sent on her own strange path, but the journey of Darnella Wilson—eighteen, naïve, and inexperienced—shows just how bad it could be.

When Freedom House was still around, Darnella was the last one in. She graduated high school in the spring of '75, and a few weeks later Walt Brown changed her life forever. One afternoon during the interlude between high school and college, her last hazy summer, Darnella was relaxing on her sister's couch when Walt Brown came in. He and her sister were friends, and when Walt saw Darnella sitting there, he asked what her plans for the summer were. Darnella had none. For a few months she had nothing to do, nowhere to go, and she intended to enjoy it. But Walt had other ideas. He knew Darnella wanted to go into medicine, and Walt being Walt, he pointed a finger at the reclined form on the couch and barked, "You need a job." She didn't want to work, but Walt ignored that. Wasn't old enough to work at Freedom House, but Walt ignored that too. Almost before she knew it, Darnella was down at Presby lying about her age on a Freedom House application.

Walt said she'd be a secretary, but that was only because he didn't know how to explain the work of a dispatcher. Darnella was hired and marched down to the base station, plopped in the seat, handed a phone. She was intimidated by the oxygen tanks and the gauze, the CPR dummies, needles, cardiac monitors, and squawking radios. The paramedics. Everyone was in their twenties, so old, and she didn't know how to act around old people. She sat hunched by the phone, so young and unworldly that she convinced herself *if I do something wrong, they're gonna tell my mom.*

But she stuck it out. Walt gave her no choice. A week in, the checks came, and Darnella was so excited to get paid that even after she spent the money, she kept the little pink stub. The money was nice, but it was everything else about Freedom House that drew her in. The equipment and the stories, calls coming in and crews rushing out, the exhilaration of a Black-run enterprise. Darnella was young and excitable, her voice bubbling over in a Pennsylvania accent, all those drawn-out vowels. The guys hung around her desk, trying to scare and impress her, to flirt with her. Then one day in walked Nancy, radio slung over her shoulder and talking to Walt. Darnella turned to the medic beside her and said, "What are y'all doing with this white woman?" Later that day she saw Nancy chew out a crew for not doing everything exactly as they should have done it, and she realized that not only was this white woman for real but the job itself was much more than trash talk and crazy stories. There was something happening here. She got interested. She talked the crews into showing her the ambulance and the gear, how to do CPR.

Walt was unimpressed. If Darnella wanted to see what they did, really see it and prove she could cut it here, the only way was to go out where the work was done. She needed to ride an ambulance. Darnella, shaking her head: "I don't know, Walt." Walt ignored that too.

"I'm the boss, and you're gonna get your little ass out there." He walked off. "Next call."

Because that's how these things work, the next call was the worst call. An old woman living in squalor. Bedridden, covered in feces. The smell so stiff you could walk on it. Darnella stopped, shook her head. *Uhn-uh. Nope. I'm outta here.* She wasn't used to the patients or the projects, and she wasn't feeling it. She wasn't even from the Hill. Darnella grew up in the nearly all-white neighborhood of Manchester in a big house with floor-length curtains and a fireplace. Her father owned a restaurant called Wilson's BBQ and threw parties attended by mayors and the well-connected, by people of means. Darnella was never sure if it was that their restaurant was so successful or their skin so light, but the Wilsons enjoyed a level of prosperity and respect foreign to her new coworkers. They didn't know her world at all and didn't care, just dragged her all the way out here to some flophouse in the Hill and—no. She was done here, thanks, ready to walk away for good when something caught her eye. It was how the medics treated this woman, how they went from being tough and cocky to so compassionate, like they didn't notice the smell.

Darnella was only a few years removed from her parents' divorce, a traumatic cleft that split up her family and took the house and the floor-length curtains in a single blow. All the things that made her feel special as a child suddenly appeared fragile—even her father's political clout was waning—and maybe Darnella, young as she was, began feeling fragile herself. Maybe she was on the lookout for something to set her apart, something more concrete than money or powerful friends, and if so, that search ended abruptly in a filthy tenement. Standing there, cotton stuffed up her nose and not wanting to touch anything, witnessing an act of grace, Darnella found her purpose in life.

And then came the end. October 15. The lights went out, and everyone danced goodbye. She turned eighteen just in time to transfer to the city, which she thought was a good thing until she found out she wasn't being hired as a dispatcher or even a secretary, but as an unarmed guard assigned to keep watch over prisoners awaiting arraignment, and really, that's when the horrors started.

ONE THING WAS quickly becoming clear: the city might've been forced to take Freedom House employees, but it wasn't forced to keep them. From the very beginning, every move seemed driven by racism and spite and aimed at weeding them out. The medics, trained to the nation's highest standards, were forced to take yet another course—administered by the city—which didn't even meet federal requirements. Even though they'd passed a more advanced version of the very same class the city's medics had taken, they were all sent back to school. Nancy was livid and protested but got nowhere. And so they sat through lectures covering topics they'd already learned and applied in the field, taught to them by instructors who were openly antagonistic and dismissive. Life was no better on the ambulance.

The medics hired by the city were told to keep an eye on the people from Freedom House because they'd been acquired not hired and had been up to God-knows-what all these years. There was a sense that anyone from Freedom House was inferior and suspect, and no amount of smiling or politeness, no pliable eagerness to please, could overcome or escape it. It was as if they had the words *FREEDOM HOUSE* tattooed across their foreheads. Overnight John went from interpreting EKGs and giving drugs, intubating patients and interacting with doctors to riding quietly in the back as an observer.

Though hired as a paramedic, he wasn't allowed to touch patients and certainly couldn't treat them—*hold the bag*. He wasn't even supposed to talk to them—*hold the bag*—which didn't matter anyway because most people went straight to the white guys, assuming them to be in charge. The message, repeated with such frequency that John almost started believing it, was that the medics from the city were better and if John, lowly as he was, kept quiet and learned, then someday he'd get there too. Maybe.

And yet, whatever (over)confidence the city medics exhibited when dealing with John disappeared the moment they rolled into the Hill. The Hill was a place they knew only from reading the papers or watching TV. They expected crime and murder, utter madness, and they showed up edgy and secretly armed with knives, brass knuckles, nunchucks—anything to beat back the menace. To them, places like the Bedford Dwellings weren't residential areas or even housing projects but war zones that required constant vigilance. A mushrooming sense of unease would set in as they approached. Still en route? Double parking at night? Doesn't matter. Kill the sirens, flip off the lights. Sneak in. They emerged from the ambulance—armed with Maglites, double-checking that the doors were locked—like Pilgrims stepping onto foreign soil. They entered slowly, without a word. *Quiet on the stairs, or they'll hear you coming.*

Try as he might, John couldn't get them to relax. Their mindset was all wrong, he told them. Dressed in city uniforms, driven by fear and prejudice and an outsized view of their own authority, the city medics looked and acted just like cops. Imagine a paramedic scolding drivers for a moving violation. It happened. Meanwhile, patients with chest pain or shortness of breath were made to get up and walk to the ambulance, and others, less acute, were told to take a jitney to the hospital. A community that had known Freedom House, that was used to getting the raw end but for eight years got the best street medicine available anywhere, struggled to adjust to this new reality. One night, Raynovich returned to his ambulance to find the windows broken out.

Whatever shortcomings the city's new service or its medics had, it was the Freedom House personnel who were treated like the problem. In addition to the course that they alone were forced to take, the Freedom House medics were singled out to sit for tests every week. Each one was forty-five minutes long and strictly pass/fail. Fail, and you were gone. Some, like John, put up with it. Some people, pushed as far as they could be pushed, simply walked away. Nancy fought for the medics as hard as she could but met resistance at every turn. Unable to be as hands-on as she would've liked, barred from directing and refining the service's standard of care, she eventually quit and turned her attention full-time to writing the paramedic training manual. In a letter to Phil Hallen, attorney Aims Coney wrote that the "city never accepted the principal of a strong, independent medical command," so "Dr. Caroline left the program in disappointment." As for the medics, Coney, whose involvement with Freedom House went back to the very beginning, said the "personnel who transferred to the city found a lack of the standards and the mission which had characterized Freedom House."

For Darnella Wilson, it was more than just a lack of standards. Her new job in the city jail was a living hell. She had just turned eighteen and now spent hours every day with incarcerated men, alone and separated only by a set of bars. The things they said to her, what she saw, it was horrible and traumatizing, and decades later she wouldn't be able to talk about it without breaking down. But she didn't give in.

The further Darnella was pushed, the more intractable she became. She enrolled in business school (just to have a backup) but stayed on at the jail out of pure defiance. All day she kept her nose in a book to keep from seeing what was happening just a few feet away, and it was hard, but she hung on until eventually she snagged a spot in the Pittsburgh EMS dispatch center. Once there, she started working her way toward the ambulance. She fought, and she clawed; she studied, prepared, and steeled herself. She refused to go away.

But not everyone was able to hang on. The classes and testing, the inability to lay hands on patients, being regarded and treated like something lowly, it all added up to beat many of the old Freedom House staff into submission. Within that first year, about half of the people who came over to Pittsburgh EMS left. One by one they walked out the door, some to other services, others to different work entirely. One became a garbage man, another a tow truck driver. Ron Ragin, part of the original class and perhaps the most experienced and talented medic in the city, struggled with the tests and was fired. He took a job with South Hills EMS but at some point left and fell off the radar, bouncing from house to house until, finally, he landed on the streets.

Then McCary got fired. Smiling George McCary, the guy who joined Freedom House after his grandmother threatened to kick him out (and who finished the course just to prove he could), the self-described hustler who knew everyone and never got flustered, the guy who helped John settle into his career, his friend and opposite, into whose hands John placed his trust and his life—his *partner*—failed a test, and he was gone. George was one of those guys who's great on a call but less so on paper, and eventually, while tiptoeing along the uninterrupted line of tests, he tripped. This one hurt. John owed something to George he couldn't repay, but there was only so much grieving he could do. They were spread out all over the city and hardly saw each other, and besides, John, too, was in survival mode. He was under the same pressure as everyone else and woke each morning with the same thought: *they're trying to fire me next*.

For John and Darnella, for everyone still hanging on, this whispered fact provided the anger and the determination to stay. The more the city wanted them gone, the harder they fought to remain. Survival became an act of resistance. They formed study groups; John hosted several sessions at his house to go over everything that could possibly be on the test. They practiced scenarios, drilled each other on anatomy and cardiology and pharmacology; they made sure anyone lagging behind was brought up to speed. They all passed. Then they passed again, and again, and they kept passing until at last the testing stopped.

But there was always something else. One day the medics—everyone this time—were put in a van and driven to a bridge. John stood on the span and looked out over the city. A brisk wind blew across his face as an instructor went over the nuances of knots and harnesses and the tricky art of rappelling from great heights.

"Okay," the instructor told him. "Climb over the railing and lean from the edge."

"The what now?"

All along John thought his job was to stop seizures and deliver babies, but here he was on a bridge with people trying to pry his fingers off the railing. Ultimately, he overcame his fear and did it, not because he wanted to—though, frankly, it wasn't that bad—but because he had to, and whether or not this had anything at all to do with medicine (it didn't), he wasn't going to quit. So he rappelled all the way to the bottom, then went up and did it again.

But you can't rappel your way into acceptance. There's no knot you can tie or course you can take, no test you can pass. The only way to get respect from someone who doesn't want to give it is to walk right over and take it.

CHAPTER FORTY-ONE

It felt like the old days all over again. Like when he was in the orphanage or newly arrived in Pittsburgh, or really at any number of points along the way where John found himself alone and out of control. Those weren't good days, and he wasn't eager to relive them, but if he had to, at least they'd taught him something about himself, about his ability to find something deep inside he didn't know was there. He needed that now. That singularity of purpose, that ability to block out the world and focus solely on his own survival.

Still, he wanted to do more than just endure. He wanted to break through. He tried any combination of polite and deferential and cooperative, but still they looked down on him. As if there was some proof he hadn't yet provided. Only he was done trying to prove himself. He was enough, and it was time they saw it, though how or when or if that would happen, he didn't know.

Until, one day, the radio crackled to life.

FAMILIAR SOUNDS. SIRENS screaming, tires humming, the dispatcher's voice—tight with anxiety—filling the air. A middle-aged man was down and possibly not breathing in Beechview, a suburban neighborhood just south of Mount Washington on the west side of town. They pulled up, and John instinctively hopped from the back and was headed for the door when one of the medics placed his hand on John's chest to stop him. *Grab the bag.*

He was loaded down with gear as the other two medics rushed to the patient's side. The man was in his fifties, on the couch and not moving. They tried to wake him but couldn't. Crouching, one of the medics checked for a pulse but found none. Standing in the back with the family, John saw what was about to happen almost before the medics themselves did. He recognized it in their posture, their voices, in the shifty way their eyes darted back and forth as they slowly did the math on the problem before them—this was their first cardiac arrest, and they were panicking.

Are you kidding me right now?, John was thinking. $35,000 dollar truck and all this equipment, the training, that smug attitude, and you're panicking? It's one thing to go to school and learn CPR, to trot out mannikins and sit through lectures, but it's something else entirely to actually do it. To be faced with a person whose life you either will or won't save. All that knowledge and the only thing that matters is whether you can put it to use. McCary, who'd been deemed unfit and was no longer there, showed him that. In those quick first seconds John wondered what to do. Watch? Step in? Give advice—*maybe we should rappel down the chimney.* For months they'd kept him in the back, a servant and not a provider. Hadn't let him do a thing. They treated him as if he was useless or worse, but now it was their first cardiac arrest, and they were panicking. When the shock wore off and they turned to him, faces white with terror, it was in both surrender and recognition. John waited, and finally one of them yelled it.

"Do something!"

And it was really that simple. The tables turned, his worth acknowledged. John snapped a finger. "You, start CPR. You, get an IV." John connected their monitor, interpreted the rhythm, and shocked the patient. Then he intubated the guy because he wasn't just someone who'd sat through a paramedic course: he was a Freedom House paramedic, heir to Peter Safar's legacy, student of the woman who literally wrote the book on prehospital medicine, a trained professional who never let anything get in the way of saving lives. And when everything was done and the patient as stabilized as he was going to get, John told the other medics to load him in the ambulance and drive to the hospital—*slowly, don't throw me around*.

That call was his breakthrough, and from that moment on he took over. He got louder and more aggressive, and instead of walking in last and letting them lead, from then on John called the shots. The victory was as contagious as it was liberating. One by one Raynovich and the others began stepping up and taking over, flexing their knowledge and experience until, by the end of the year, the guys from Freedom House ceased being the guys from Freedom House and were seen as the one thing all along they knew themselves to be: paramedics.

EPILOGUE

A constant clack of typewriter keys. Nancy shivering in the frigid air that seeped through the walls of her apartment. Another season of discontent. It was winter (again), 1975.

The class she taught back in the spring, the one that propelled John and the rest of the Freedom House paramedics back to the forefront of street medicine, had been embraced by the US Department of Transportation and would soon become the official paramedic curriculum taught in over forty states. She now had a contract to transform the entire experience—all those hours in the classroom, the *let's-just-sneak-in-here* lab time, every night she'd spent speeding through the streets—into a first-of-its-kind paramedic training textbook. It sounded like a good idea when she'd first been approached by the publisher, Little, Brown, but now that she actually had to create the textbook, on top of her job as medical director to Pittsburgh EMS, plus her duties as assistant professor of clinical anesthesiology and critical care medicine at the University of Pittsburgh, well, it was almost too much. Maybe it actually was too much—Nancy was so buried in work she didn't have time to take stock of just how busy she actually was.

She was back to not sleeping.

It'd been only a year since she agreed to join Freedom House, but that year had been so full—of work, of frustration, of tragedy, of loss and elation, of life—it must surely have felt like ten. She wanted to rest now but couldn't. And so she typed, bent over a typewriter in an apartment so cold that her cousin Audrey loaned her an electric space heater just so she wouldn't freeze to death. The gesture backfired. When Nancy plugged it in, the fuses in her apartment blew, and the whole place went dark. She went down to the basement, tinkered with the fuse box until she figured out how to replace the broken ones, then trudged back up to her apartment only to find that she'd locked herself out.

The next year, 1976, brought no relief. In June she left Pittsburgh EMS in frustration. Needing a clean break, Nancy resigned from her position at the University of Pittsburgh and accepted a job nearby as deputy director of the Emergency Department at Shadyside Hospital. She did what she could to maintain her ties with the people of Freedom House but not even all their shared history—and history making—could hold them together. One by one the eighty-plus people who at one time or another worked at Freedom House went on to different, and quite often bigger, things.

By October 1976, only twelve of the twenty-six Freedom House personnel who went over to the city remained there. John Bucci and John Barnett, Will Holland, James Kyte, David Lindell and Tim Payer, Craig Simmons—they all remained on as paramedics with the city. So did Irv Davis and Eugene Key. Within a couple years both would be promoted to supervisor. Darnella Wilson fought through her ordeal at the jail to become a paramedic. She stayed on with Pittsburgh EMS for thirty-five years and eventually got her nursing degree. She's also a noted jazz singer who sang the national anthem at a Pittsburgh Steelers game and once performed in Manhattan with trumpet legend Freddie Hubbard.

Raynovich was another one who survived the transition. He stayed with the city until 1983, then served as liaison between officials at McKeesport Hospital and local EMS companies, and eventually became director of the University of New Mexico EMS Academy. Walt Brown became paramedic coordinator at the University Health Center's Department of Anesthesiology. Dave Rayzer earned a PhD in public health. Gerald Esposito, the man who once ran an ambulance company out of his kitchen and had been a part of Freedom House's support staff since the very beginning, became executive director of the Emergency Medical Services Institute in southwest Pennsylvania.

Others left medicine altogether. William Draper moved on. So did David Clemons. Kerry Muckle became an insurance agent. After leaving the city, George McCary got a job as a cab driver and later wrote to Nancy, "I have wisely used the time to find myself." Found, perhaps, but not changed. He chatted up everyone he met and was quick to point out just who it was sitting up front driving the cab. "You can't say you [met] the first doctor, and you [met] the first police officer," he'd tell his fares. "But you can say you met one of the first American, worldwide EMT paramedics."

Mitch Brown became paramedic training coordinator for the EMS Operations Center at the University of Pittsburgh. In 1980 he moved to Cleveland, where he took over the EMS department, immediately butting heads with the fire chief over Mitch's plans to create a paramedic training institute and upgrade the service to advanced life support. When the chief pushed back, saying he already had the best people around, Mitch said, "Well, you call the best person you got and get them here, and I'll embarrass him or her right in front of you."

So, the ALS upgrade went on as planned. Six years later Mitch was promoted to Cleveland's public safety director. In April 2000 he was hired to do the same job in Columbus. In 2016, he was appointed to a vacant seat on the Columbus City Council and won election the following year. He retired in 2021.

Phil Hallen remained at the Falk Medical Fund for the rest of his career. In 2000, shortly before he retired, the University of Pittsburgh honored his thirty-five years of service to the city by endowing the Phil Hallen Chair in Community Health and Social Justice.

Even as everyone from this period of his life moved on to other endeavors, other places, Peter Safar remained at Pitt. Eva once described their life together as living in the eye of a hurricane. His frenetic activity didn't stop. In 1979 he stepped down as head of anesthesiology to create yet another department within the university health system. The International Resuscitation Research Center, renamed the Safar Center in 1994, took Safar's critical care and CPR work a step further. Among other advances, the Center pioneered resuscitative hypothermia—a rapid cooling of the body—which buys time for doctors trying to save a patient by preserving brain tissue in the event of sudden death. For this work, Safar would be nominated three times (1990, 1992, and 1994) for the Nobel Prize in Medicine.

In later years, he lamented the rise of bureaucrats who hindered the advance of medical innovation, and also the steady creep of commerce into what had been a collegial field. He remained altruistic but admitted sometimes he took the idea too far. He'd resisted efforts, for instance, by Johnson & Johnson to patent the S-tube he developed to assist with mouth-to-mouth, and though he had a hand in creating it, Safar never asked for, nor received, any money from Asmund Laerdal for sales of the Resusci Annie doll, on which hundreds of millions of people were trained in CPR. (As a strange aside, Annie's face was modeled after a young woman who in the late nineteenth century drowned in the Seine. When no one claimed her, she was put on display but never identified. Yet her smile, even in death, was so enigmatic, so strangely Mona Lisa, it captivated Paris, and thousands of plaster casts of her face were sold. One of these death masks hung in the home of Laerdal's grandparents.)

Safar continued working, continued traveling and playing music with Eva, continued plotting, until his death in August 2003 at the age of seventy-nine. He lived a life as full as a Russian epic, big gambles and bigger ideas, always in motion. Among the few constants was his friendship with Nancy.

In 1977, Nancy realized her childhood ambition of living in Israel when she accepted a position as EMS director for Magen David Adom, Israel's national disaster response agency. At the time, MDA fielded ambulance techs but had no paramedic program. Nancy was recruited to do for Israel's ambulance service what she'd done at Freedom House. It wasn't an easy task. As had been the case in the United States, there was official resistance to creating a paramedic program, and Nancy, an American, was received by some with skepticism. She didn't even know Hebrew and instead relied on a secretary who translated everything happening around her. If she was in any way overwhelmed by the task, she didn't let it show. Armed with her unpublished training textbook—*Emergency Care in the Streets* wouldn't be released until January 1979—she trained and then supervised the country's first paramedics.

As in Pittsburgh, Nancy couldn't be confined to the classroom. On March 11, 1978, militants from the Palestinian Liberation Organization attacked a bus on the road between Haifa and Tel Aviv. Nancy arrived with the first wave of ambulances, only to be pinned down by automatic rifle fire. She was forced to watch as the crowded bus burned. This incident sparked further hostilities between Israel and the PLO along the Lebanese border, and Nancy was repeatedly dispatched to an MDA aid station in Metula, a sliver of land on the border with Lebanon, to treat civilian casualties. Despite the danger, she was taken with the town and its fragrant orange groves and eventually moved there.

In 1982 she decamped for Nairobi, where she worked as one of the famed "flying doctors" of the African Medical and Research Foundation. For the next five years, Nancy trained health care workers and treated patients in Kenya, Tanzania, Uganda, and Sudan, covering a quarter of a million miles of east Africa in a small plane. She wrote a weekly column in the Kenyan newspaper, the *Standard*, called "Ask Dr. AMREF," became a global leader in the burgeoning field of disaster medicine, and started an agricultural nonprofit to combat food shortages.

In 1987 she returned to Israel, where her renovated house in Metula was hit three times by rockets. She wrote to Safar that she was conscripted into joining night patrols, "presumably looking for terrorists . . . though I'm not sure I'd recognize [a terrorist] if I tripped over one."

Nancy dedicated the rest of her career to first creating, then expanding, the field of palliative care in Israel and, in 1995, founded Hospice of the Upper Galilee, which continues operating today. In 2002 she married the geneticist and molecular biologist Lazarus Astrachan, whom she'd met in medical school. If the goal was to settle down at last, fate intervened. The same year Nancy and Astrachan married, she was diagnosed with multiple myeloma. Knowing she was terminal, Nancy returned to Boston to visit her mother one final time. She was escorted back to the States by a contingent of Israeli paramedics, who carried her bags and ensured she was comfortable, a final nod of respect to the woman they'd come to know as "Israel's Mother Teresa." Dr. Nancy Caroline spent her final days in her own hospice center and died on December 12, 2002.

WHATEVER ACHIEVEMENTS OR adventure Nancy found around the world, her mind was never far from the Hill. Years after leaving Pittsburgh, she wrote how the distant wail of a siren still evoked a "peculiar bond with remote events, a sense of shared experience: I was part of this too." Exactly what it was she'd been a part of, in the years after Freedom House closed down, seemed in some ways an open question. It was sometimes referred to as a pilot program or an experiment, as if it'd been nothing but a dry run for all the EMS advances that followed. But even this passing recognition faded, and by the mid-'80s Freedom House wasn't mentioned at all.

This gradual forgetting continued even as the forces that'd once been aligned against them disappeared. Police departments and funeral homes were forced out of the ambulance business. As for Flaherty, after his second term as mayor, he launched three unsuccessful campaigns—two for the US Senate and one for governor. He served briefly in the Justice Department under President Jimmy Carter and ended his political career with a short stint as county commissioner. William Hunt lost his seat on the County Commission in 1983 to fellow Republican Barbara Hafer, who drew strong support after Hunt referred to her as "the little nurse from Elizabeth."

As the world moved on, the medics themselves, though to a lesser degree, were doing the same. Even John.

He survived the transition and stayed on at Pittsburgh EMS. For the next two years he rode a city ambulance, waiting, as he had back at the steel mill, for the day when someone would see his potential and lift him up into the ranks of management. It didn't happen. And so in 1977 he walked into Cannon's office and demanded to know why. He was experienced, reliable, and highly competent. He was a crew chief and had as much time on the streets as almost anybody. John laid out his case and then (to Cannon's apparent surprise) made a simple demand. When the next slot came open, it had to be his.

And it was.

John's parents, never entirely certain what this wayward son of theirs did for a living, swelled with pride when they learned he was a supervisor. John worked hard to live up to the post. He tried to be fair, to be helpful. He kept his truck clean and his uniform impeccable. The beard was gone, and slowly, over time, the afro went away too. He was older but still young, and had already pulled himself through enough trouble for two lifetimes. He wasn't always perfect. The self-reliance that so often carried him through hardship took its toll on his marriage. He and Betty separated and would ultimately divorce.

But he tried not to look back and rarely did he think about the old days anymore. Unless a song came on. "Lonely Teardrops" could set him right down in another time. Mostly, though, he let himself forget. The '60s and the '70s, hope and rebellion and all the heartache that came with it, even Freedom House. People didn't want to talk about it. So he didn't.

Then came that day in 1984, the call for a man screaming at the intersection of Fifth and Market, and the memories came flooding back. The next part you know. John pulling up to find Ragin, his old friend, one of the very first paramedics, maybe the best of them—his mind all but gone—surrounded by cops every bit as scared and uncertain and angry. The potential in that moment, with police officers dispatched to deal with a psychiatric emergency, for everything to go terribly and irrevocably wrong.

What happened that day, seeing Ragin on the street, it got him thinking. About how the problems he had with the cops back in the '60s and '70s still existed (in 1997 Pittsburgh would become the first city to enter into a consent decree with the Department of Justice over issues of police misconduct). How the EMS department was now almost entirely white even though its roots were in the Black community. And what of those roots? Ambulance design, training, equipment, standards, procedures, Nancy's paramedic textbook (still the go-to resource today) all stemmed from Freedom House, and yet hardly anybody had ever heard of it.

The names and faces, the voices of those who decades ago took a leap of faith and started a revolution that saved countless lives across the world: nobody knew them. No one heard them. Like the uprising in 1968, they were bottled up and held at bay, their voices silenced. They'd been left to slip through the cracks, and the injustice of it was reflected so perfectly in the sight of Ragin screaming in the middle of the street less than a decade after the end that it hit John all at once.

Years ago, Nancy had encouraged him to see the bigger picture and to carry on. No matter what. John had carried on; that much was certain. The lessons he learned when he was young, of relying on no one, of focusing strictly on his own survival, had carried him through. But they obscured the bigger picture. He made it, but others had been left behind along the way. The ultimate goal, to be heard, still lay out there. Somewhere.

Slowly, but in every way, this encounter changed John's life. He worked harder and with bigger goals. He brought others with him, helping to end a law that said you had to be part of a volunteer department before you could get hired onto a paid department by arguing that people struggling to feed their families can't afford to donate their time. He created a program within Pittsburgh EMS to recruit students from low-income neighborhoods, send them to EMT school, and then offer them a job. And he fought to keep Freedom House alive.

In 2002, he successfully petitioned to have historical decals commemorating Freedom House placed on all the ambulances in the city, and then, a few years later, when new ambulances came out—without the decals—he started pushing again. He also joined his old coworkers in successful efforts to have a commemorative plaque placed at Presby. In 2004 he was promoted to assistant chief. Even after retiring in 2009, he carried on the fight. He talked about Freedom House nonstop. He traveled the country; he went on radio and TV and answered every call from every reporter—there weren't many—who called to see what it'd all been about. In 2019, Amera Gilchrist became the first woman and first Black person promoted to the rank of deputy chief of Pittsburgh EMS. After her promotion, Deputy Chief Gilchrist said, "Mr. Moon was instrumental in getting me to this place."

That, more than anything, is the lasting legacy of Freedom House. The lives saved and the lives inspired by people who rose up from the ashes of their own smoldering neighborhood to answer cries for help. It's been a long struggle for recognition, far from over, but to the question of whether it was all worth it, Darnella has a simple answer: "Hell yeah."

John, in his own way, says the same. And so he's still out there. The glasses are thicker. And he drives a Cadillac instead of an ambulance. But he talks about it. About Freedom House and how the lessons and techniques developed there, the course, Nancy's textbook (now in its eighth edition) inspired everything that came after. How the birth of the paramedic—in which they played a critical role—changed the way Americans live and die. But mostly he talks about the people who answered the call to help. How they did it because it was the right thing to do but also to show people they could.

On the day John was called out to help Ragin, after he channeled the spirit of George McCary—an easy voice, a little charm—to defuse an explosive situation, the two old friends sat on the wall and, eventually, after Ragin relaxed, started talking. About ambulances and emergencies, about all those years they spent in the base station and Presby, in the Bedford Dwellings. About running calls in back alleys and restaurants. They talked about Freedom House, which really meant talking about the people. Safar and Nancy, Walt, Mitch, George, everybody they once knew so well but no longer. It brought them back in time, to *that* time. The moment they changed everything. And if you'd been there that day to listen, even if you asked him now what they said, that's what John would tell you. What he'd want you to know. That they were here, and maybe they're gone, but they'd like you to remember them. Their names, their faces, their voices. They would like to be heard. They've waited a long time to share their story, and perhaps now, after all these years, the rest of us are finally ready to listen.

In Pittsburgh, in 1966, twenty-four Black men from the Hill answered a call for help and in the process changed the world. They were sons and fathers, bookbinders, mechanics, orderlies. They were paramedics, and they came from Freedom House. *Freedom House. Now I know you remember that.* They did something truly remarkable, for that or any other time, and their story goes something like this. . . .

MEMBERS OF FREEDOM HOUSE AMBULANCE SERVICE

(in alphabetical order)

Michael Blackman*
Nancy Brandon (dispatcher)
Harold Brown*
Jules Brown
Mitchell Brown*
Walter Brown*
Barbara Bryant (dispatcher)
John Bucci
John Burnett
Gary Burnworth
Issac Camp
Glenn Cannon
Barbara Carter (dispatcher)
David Clemens*
Tom Clowney
Arthur Davis*
Irv Davis
Ray Davis*
Rhonda Davis (secretary)
Dianne Denning (secretary)
Dennis Ditley
William Draper

Virgil Duckett
Clyde Dunson*
John Franklin*
Harvey Gandy*
Paul Garnes
Tom Geier
Tom Grace*
Lonnie Green III
Donna Griffith (dispatcher)
Darlene Griggs (dispatcher)
Harry Harrison
Joe Hirsch
Gary Hitchings
Harold Holland*
Will Holland
Pat Hollyfield (dispatcher)
Marshall Hornstein
Addie Johnson*
Ruth Johnson (dispatcher)
Eugene Key*
James Kyte*
Vernon Lane
Shelly Lewis (secretary)
David Lindell
Toni Long (secretary)
Jean Madosky (dispatcher)
Eugene Marks
Frank Mascaro
George McCary*
William McDoodle
George Mitchell

Thomas Mitchell*
John Moon
Wilma Mosely (dispatcher)
Kerry Muckler
Daniel Nickens*
Rick Orange
Deborah Owens (dispatcher)
Doris Owens (dispatcher)
Tim Payer
Pearl Porter (dispatcher)
William Porter*
Tom Preston
Raymond Pridgen*
Ron Ragin*
William Raynovich
David Rayzer*
Calvin Richardson
Lorraine Saffer (dispatcher)
Curtis Scott*
Craig Simmons
Ernest Simpson*
Carl Staten*
Wallace Sullivan*
David Thomas*
Thomas Wade*
Kenneth Williams*
Darnella Wilson (dispatcher)

* *indicates member of the first two training classes, 1967–1968*

ACKNOWLEDGMENTS

This book is the culmination of three years of work, prompted by an unsolicited text that included a few lines about something called Freedom House and the (seemingly) innocuous question "Have you ever heard of these guys?"

Sadly, I had not. Though I'd spent a decade of my life as a paramedic, an experience I turned into a book and many episodes of television, I was wholly unaware (as were nearly every single one of my coworkers) of the men and women whose dedication and professionalism had produced so many of the things in my ambulance that I took for granted. That single text message stirred my curiosity. I spent an afternoon online that, by dusk, produced a name that would change my life: John Moon.

By now I know John, as I hope you do, but back then, in 2018, I had no idea who he was and little sense of what he'd done or first had to overcome in order to do it. Nor did John know anything about me. To him I was just another stranger calling to ask about that time, all those years ago, when he helped to change the world. But he took the call and patiently laid out for me the bones of a truly remarkable story. And he kept telling that story, day after day, over the years, answering each time I called (which was too many times to count), never tiring, even of me as far as I could tell. Each time my name popped up on the screen of his cell phone, whether he was at home or the grocery store, he'd answer with a pleasant "Well, hey Kevin, how you doing?" Why he did this, aside from being a truly kind and generous man, was that he never lost faith either in the power of his story or that one day the world would care enough to hear it. He told me, way back during that first call, that Freedom House wasn't a job but a calling, that it had saved him and given him purpose and pride, and for that, and a million other reasons, he owed the service and everyone who ever wore the uniform a debt he can never repay. That's exactly how the rest of us—certainly the world's paramedics, undeniably me—should feel about him. John, along with everyone at Freedom House, quite literally saved us, at a bargain rate of just a few dollars an hour. He's given generations of medics purpose and pride. At a time when I genuinely needed it, he gave me a renewed faith in humanity, not to mention the story of a lifetime. I couldn't have written this book without John. His time, his patience, his candor while entrusting me with what surely were painful memories, all in the name of getting this story out, were truly inspiring. John, in a time when heroes are in short supply, you fit the bill quite nicely. I thank you, my friend, from the bottom of my heart.

I'd like to thank everyone who took the time to share their stories with me: Phil Hallen, Darnella Wilson, Bill Raynovich, George McCary, and Mitch Brown. Peter Caroline, who shared stories of growing up with Nancy, and Oren Wacht, who filled in the blanks of Nancy's time in Israel. Fran Mistrick, who opened up about what it was like to have Peter Safar as a boss; Paul Safar, who shared what it was like to have him as a father; and Eva (she took my call even as a wildfire forced her to evacuate), who told me what it was like to share a life with him. Robert Clinchy, who provided key information about the early days of EMS, and Kris Cagle, my own paramedic instructor, who opened my eyes to the horrors and hilarity of providing emergency care from the back of a hearse.

A special thanks to Jonah Ogles, who shared my passion for this story from day one and expertly edited a version of it for the *Atavist* magazine, and Seyward Darby, whose steady hand guided us over the finish line. A huge thanks to Roman Mars, Joe Rosenberg, Delaney

Hall, and everyone at *99% Invisible* for shepherding me through the podcast process.

This book might not have happened at all if my agent and sounding board/part-time shrink, Alice Martell, hadn't called and insisted that I give this story one last shot after I'd hit a wall and nearly shelved the project. And it certainly would not be in the shape it's in now had it not been for Sam Raim, editor extraordinaire, who got the pitch at nine a.m. and offered to buy it at a little past noon. Thank you both: I am indebted beyond my ability to pay.

To my wife, who endured my absences and grumpiness, who listened as I searched for a way to turn years of research into a coherent story and then read (and reread) the results, and who, quite generously, turned her favorite room in our house into my office, thank you is never enough.

Finally, to everyone who ever picked up a shift on a Freedom House ambulance, a grateful nation sends its thanks.

NOTES

PROLOGUE

xix **Ragin screaming:** Phone interviews with John Moon, 2020–2021.

xix **overrun by crime:** "Pittsburgh's Market Square Constantly Changes, but Its Purpose Hasn't Wavered Since 1784," *Incline*, August 14, 2018, archive.theincline.com/2018/08/14/pittsburghs-market-square-constantly-changes-but-its-purpose-hasnt-wavered-since-1784; editorial, *Pittsburgh Post-Gazette*, May 8, 1984, 4.

xix **Across town:** Phone interviews with John Moon, 2020.

xx **Ragin had peered over:** Ibid.; phone interview with Darnella Wilson, August 2020.

xx **next to an oyster house:** "Sites of the Underground Railroad," Visit Pittsburgh, www.visitpittsburgh.com/things-to-do/arts-culture/history/underground-railroad, accessed February 1, 2022.

xxi **Market Square tingled:** Phone interviews with John Moon, 2020.

xxi **trying to drag him to the ground:** Phone interview with John Moon, November 2021.

xxi **"I know him:** Ibid.

xxii **some forty-four students:** D. M. Benson, G. Esposito, J. Dirsch, et al., "Mobile Intensive Care by 'Unemployable' Blacks Trained as Emergency Medical Technicians (EMT's) in 1967–69," *Journal of Trauma* 12, no. 5 (1972): 408–421.

xxiii **Ragin had been one:** Freedom House employee rolls, from the Papers of Nancy L. Caroline, 1905–2007, Schlesinger Library, Radcliffe Institute, Harvard University.

xxiii **"Want a job:** Joe W. Trotter and Jared N. Day, *Race and Renaissance: African Americans in Pittsburgh Since World War II* (Pittsburgh: University of Pittsburgh Press, 2010), 113.

xxiv **For Ragin, maybe the best:** Phone interviews with John Moon, 2020.

CHAPTER ONE

2 **"Hospital orderly.":** In-person interview with John Moon, April 2019.

3 **"Mr. Smith,":** Ibid.

4 **"Those were *Black* guys.":** Ibid.

5 **almost all of whom were Black:** Phone interview with John Moon, December 2021.

5 ***They're known for stealing things*:** In-person interview with John Moon, April 2019.

6 **Two weeks later:** Ibid.

CHAPTER TWO

10 **John Moon was born:** Phone interview with John Moon, August 2018.

10 **even after its 1965 integration:** Brendan P. Lovasik, Priya R. Rajdev, Steven C. Kim, et al., "The Living Monument: The Desegregation of Grady Memorial Hospital and the Changing South," *American Surgeon* 86, no. 3 (March 2020): 213–219.

10 **It has always sat in the historic heart:** "Alonzo Herndon, Atlanta's First Black Millionaire," *Atlanta Journal-Constitution*, February 17, 2016.

10 **It was a mid-twentieth-century urban:** "Atlanta's Buttermilk Bottom," The Smithsonian's National Museum of African American Culture, February 13, 2010, web.archive.org/web/20100609172009/http:/nmaahc.si.edu/memory/view/138.

11 **Occasionally, because they could:** Ibid.

11 **Wedged alongside them:** "25Pt. of City's Houses Located in Slum Sections," *Atlanta Constitution*, July 25, 1955, 19.

11 **So it was Elzora:** In-person interview with John Moon, April 2019.

11 **"Long as I'm not working,":** Ibid.

12 **The cops came a lot:** Ibid.

13 **It happened in October 1956:** In-person interview with John Moon, April 2019; *Atlanta Constitution*, October 17, 1956, 32.

13 **Hanley's Bell Street Funeral Home:** *Atlanta Constitution*, April 8, 1968.

14 **What followed was hazy:** In-person interview with John Moon, April 2019.

14 **"Ain't no negotiating,":** Phone interview with John Moon, March 2019.

14 **Just a few years later, in 1962:** Digital Scholarship Lab, "Renewing Inequality: Urban Renewal, Family Displacements, and Race 1955–1966,"

American Panorama, ed. Robert K. Nelson and Edward L. Ayers, dsl .richmond.edu/panorama/renewal, accessed February 1, 2022.

15 **New York City got:** Ibid.

16 **By the early '60s:** Ibid.

16 **In Southern California:** "Chávez Ravine: A Los Angeles Story," Zinn Education Project, www.zinnedproject.org/materials/chavez-ravine, accessed March 4, 2022.

16 **"Urban renewal . . . :** "A Conversation with James Baldwin," televised interview with Dr. Kenneth Clark, May 24, 1963.

16 **Afterward, Baldwin was scheduled:** "An Interview with Author James Baldwin," Open Vault, WGBH Archives, April 2012, openvault.wgbh .org/about.

17 **In Philadelphia and Detroit:** Digital Scholarship Lab, "Renewing Inequality: Urban Renewal, Family Displacements, and Race 1955–1966, *American Panorama*, ed. Robert K. Nelson and Edward L. Ayers, dsl .richmond.edu/panorama/renewal, accessed February 1, 2022.

17 **Overcrowding was so bad:** Ibid.

17 **the 1966 Hough Riots:** "Hough Riots," *Encyclopedia of Cleveland History*, Case Western Reserve University, case.edu/ech/articles/h /hough-riots, accessed March 4, 2022; "The Hough Uprisings of 1966," Cleveland Historical, clevelandhistorical.org/items/show/7, accessed March 4, 2022.

17 **Back in Atlanta:** "How Atlanta Displaces Black Families for Short-Term Projects," Atlanta Progressive News, April 3, 2014, atlantapro gressivenews.com/2014/04/03/analysis-how-atlanta-displaces-black -families-for-short-term-projects.

18 **"Now we're talking about:** A Conversation with James Baldwin."

18 **The stress of it:** In-person interview with John Moon, April 2019.

19 **"Get in the truck.":** Ibid.

19 **"Your father's gonna talk:** Phone interview with John Moon, May 2019.

20 **That's when the panic set in:** Ibid.

CHAPTER THREE

21 **particularly hard on June:** Phone interview with John Moon, May 2019.

21 **The orphanage had a claustrophobic:** Ibid.

22 **the kids lived on emotional islands:** Phone interview with John Moon, August 2020.

22 **"I got thirty other kids:** Ibid.

23 **"Your father died.":** Ibid.

24 **it felt like magic:** Phone interview with John Moon, September 2020.

25 **"I'm going to adopt you.":** In-person interview with John Moon, April 2019.

CHAPTER FOUR

26 **What in their minds:** Phone interview with John Moon, August 2020.

27 **The decision to adopt:** Ibid.

27 **Once it got underway:** Ibid.

28 **He hadn't been hugged:** In-person interview with John Moon, April 2019.

29 **He was angry:** Ibid.

29 **The details of how she'd died:** Phone interview with John Moon, August 2020.

CHAPTER FIVE

31 **Basically never wore:** In-person interview with John Moon, April 2019.

32 **Once owned by the grandson:** "Hill District: Crossroads of the World," Pittsburgh Music History, sites.google.com/site/pittsburghmusichistory/pittsburgh-music-story/jazz/hill-district, accessed March 4, 2022.

32 **It was home to the *Pittsburgh Courier*:** "The History of the New Pittsburgh Courier," *New Pittsburgh Courier*, newpittsburghcourier.com/the-history-of-the-new-pittsburgh-courier, accessed March 4, 2022.

32 **it was jazz that made:** Trotter and Day, *Race and Renaissance*, 22.

33 **Slumlords owned much:** "Traces of a Lost Neighborhood," *Pittsburgh Post-Gazette*, June 18, 2018.

33 **The Hill was the sort of place:** Phone interview with John Moon, January 2019.

33 **In the 1950s, Pittsburgh:** "Traces of a Lost Neighborhood."

33 **"There would be no social loss:** "Hill District: Crossroads of the World."

33 **The architect of Pittsburgh's:** "Traces of a Lost Neighborhood."

33 **The Hill's Black leadership:** Ibid.

33 **Tuberculosis and pneumonia rates:** Mark Whitaker, *Smoketown: The Other Great Black Renaissance* (New York: Simon & Schuster, 2018), 316.

34 **"Mississippi of the North":** Trotter and Day, *Race and Renaissance*, 48.

34 **"take a white man:** Ibid., 49–50.

34 **Work officially began:** Whitaker, *Smoketown*, 318–319.

34 **The Crosstown Boulevard:** "Proposed Golden Triangle—1939: 'The Moses Plan' and Point State Park," The Brookline Connection, www.brooklineconnection.com/history/Facts/Point39.html, accessed March 4, 2022.

34 **Eight thousand people:** "Traces of a Lost Neighborhood."

35 **People marched in the streets:** Trotter and Day, *Race and Renaissance*, 91–93.

CHAPTER SIX

36 **"Good evening,":** *CBS Evening News with Walter Cronkite*, April 4, 1968.

36 **Eight hundred miles away:** "The Week the Hill Rose Up," *Pittsburgh Post-Gazette*, April 2, 2018.

36 **Faculty at the Fifth:** Phone interview with John Moon, October 2018.

36 **"They killed the most:** "The Week the Hill Rose Up."

36 **A meat market:** Ibid.

36 **Just the day before:** Ibid.

37 **"They're hitting everything!":** Ibid.

37 **John was dizzy:** Phone interview with John Moon, October 2018.

37 **On day three:** Whitaker, 322.

37 **They were here to contain:** Phone interview with John Moon, October 2018.

38 **The numbers were staggering:** Whitaker, *Smoketown*, 323.

38 **"a fire in the belly.":** "The Week the Hill Rose Up."

38 **"to show that we are dissatisfied:** Letter to the Editor, *Pittsburgh Post-Gazette*, May 8, 1968.

38 **All the same:** Phone interview with John Moon, October 2018.

39 **"What white Americans:** *Report of the National Advisory Commission on Civil Disorders*, commissioned by President Lyndon B. Johnson, February 29, 1968, 1.

39 **Nevertheless, John's parents:** Phone interview with John Moon, February 2021.

39 **"Don't be doing:** Ibid.

39 **"It's a white man's world:** Ibid.

39 **His parents grew up:** Ibid.

39 **"Segregation now:** George Wallace, inaugural address, January 4, 1963.

40 **Even before the assassination:** Whitaker, *Smoketown*, 322.

CHAPTER SEVEN

41 **"It's kind of an obsession:** Phone interview with John Moon, December 2018.

42 **"Since the first time I saw:** Ibid.

42 **"You're able to identify:** Ibid.

43 **"I see.":** Ibid.

CHAPTER EIGHT

47 **Thirteenth-century Florence:** Ryan Corbett Bell, *The Ambulance: A History* (Jefferson, NC: McFarland & Co., 2009), 5–10.

47 **Dominique Jean Larrey:** Ibid., 18–21.

48 **"beyond all description":** Dr. Lindsey Fitzharris, "The Horrors of Pre-Anesthetic Surgery," July 16, 2014, www.drlindseyfitzharris.com/2014/07/16/the-horrors-of-pre-anaesthetic-surgery.

48 **So Larrey devised a solution:** Bell, *The Ambulance*, 18–21.

48 **Then came cholera:** Ibid., 24.

48 **The outbreak started:** "Cholera," History, September 12, 2017, www.history.com/topics/inventions/history-of-cholera.

48 **In its inaugural run:** Ibid.

49 **People were terrified:** "Cholera in Victorian London," Science Museum (London), July 30, 2019, www.sciencemuseum.org.uk/objects-and-stories/medicine/cholera-victorian-london.

49 **(something called Burking):** "Cholera."

49 **London's death toll:** Charles E. Rosenberg, *The Cholera Years: The United States in 1832, 1849, and 1866* (Chicago: University of Chicago Press, 1962).

49 **On January 9, 1861:** "'Star of the West' Is Fired Upon," History, November 3, 2009, www.history.com/this-day-in-history/star-of-the-west-is-fired-upon.

49 **Casualties were massive:** Bell, *The Ambulance*, 22–23.

49 **"of the lowest character.":** Ibid., 35.

50 **"The scarcity:** Ibid., 37.

50 **Heartbroken and enraged:** Ibid.

50 **"A Brief Plea for an Ambulance System.":** Ibid., 38.

50 **a man named James Jackson:** Ibid., 51.

50 **on June 4, 1869:** Ibid., 57.

51 **Alerted to an emergency:** Ibid., 60–61.

51 **In the beginning, Bellevue:** Ibid., 61–62.

51 **By the end of the year:** Ibid., 62.

52 **In 1849, Elizabeth Blackwell:** Ibid., 114.

52 **"She'll do.":** Ibid., 116.

53 **The Ford Motor Company:** "How World War I Revolutionized Medicine," *Atlantic*, February 24, 2017.

54 **Selected directly from the ranks:** John Heeg, "Stretcher-Bearers," Medicine in the First World War, History and Philosophy of Medicine, School of Medicine, University of Kansas, www.kumc.edu/school-of-medicine/academics/departments/history-and-philosophy-of-medicine/archives/wwi/essays/military-medical-operations/stretcher-bearers.html, accessed March 4, 2022.

54 **Between 1934 and 1949:** Bell, *The Ambulance*, 227.

55 **shouts of "Corpsman!":** Ibid., 241.

55 **A survey conducted a few years later:** Ibid., 245.

54 **They were short on doctors:** Ibid., 228–229.

55 **In 1965, forty-nine thousand Americans:** Bell, *The Ambulance*, 245.

56 **Highway Safety Act:** Ibid., 246.

56 **ambulance technicians were too few:** Phone interview with Richard Clinchy, August 2020.

56 **According to the White Paper:** Bell, *The Ambulance*, 250.

56 **But they never made good:** Ibid., 250.

55 **By the 1950s:** Ibid., 250.

CHAPTER NINE

58 **On the night of November 4:** Peter J. Safar, *Careers in Anesthesiology: An Autobiographical Memoir*, vol. 5: *From Pittsburgh to Vienna* (Schaumburg, IL: Wood Library-Museum of Anesthesiology, 2000), 210.

58 **However fast Safar walked:** Phone interview with Paul Safar, March 2019.

59 **Known forever-after as the Father of CPR:** "The Breath of Life" (obituary), *Detroit Metro Times*, January 7, 2004.

59 **The problem was nobody:** Safar, *Careers in Anesthesiology*, vol. 5, 206–208.

59 **Around seven thirty on the night:** "Democrat Rally Gets 'Respectable' Crowd," *Pittsburgh Post-Gazette*, November 5, 1966, 1.

60 **twenty-five hundred people in attendance:** Ibid.

60 **Despite rumblings of a rift:** "Ex-Governor Stricken at Mosque Rally," *Pittsburgh Post-Gazette*, November 5, 1966, 1.

60 **He was beloved:** "Eulogies Hail Public Servant Dave Lawrence," *Pittsburgh Press*, November 22, 1966, 4.

60 **Words like *fear*:** "Lawrence Notes Bare Unity Plea," *Pittsburgh Post-Gazette*, November 7, 1966, 2.

60 **Without warning, he toppled:** "Ex-Governor Stricken at Mosque Rally."

61 **Either that or he said:** "Lawrence Notes Bare Unity Plea."

61 **State Secretary of Internal Affairs:** "'No Chance,' Doctor Says," *Pittsburgh Press*, November 6, 1966, 4.

61 **"almost visible shock":** "Ex-Governor Stricken at Mosque Rally."

61 **Karen McGuire, a twenty-two-year-old nurse:** Ibid.

61 **Their doctrine of haste:** Bell, *The Ambulance*, 257; phone interview with Phil Hallen, February 2019; Safar, *Careers in Anesthesiology*, vol. 5, 210.

62 **the cops' cannister was either empty:** Phone interview with Phil Hallen; "Hunt, Pitt Doctor Trade Views in City Ambulance Service Battle," *Pittsburgh Press*, May 6, 1973, 22.

62 **For all intents and purposes:** "Breathing Without Aid of Machine," *Pittsburgh Press*, November 7, 1966, 1.

63 **"If we could have reached him:** Ibid.

CHAPTER TEN

64 **He was born in Vienna:** Safar, *Careers in Anesthesiology*, vol. 5, 13.

64 **They were bohemians:** Ibid.

64 **Their parents debated:** Ibid., 4.

64 **could rarely afford meat:** Ibid., 20.

64 **On March 11, 1938:** Ibid., 21.

64 **"communists . . . socialists:** Ibid.

65 **Vinca's showed that:** Ibid., 23.

65 **Karl lost his:** Ibid.

65 **At thirteen he was conscripted:** Ibid., 25.

65 **After high school:** Ibid., 30.

65 **The wet wool irritated his skin:** Ibid., 33.

65 **For the next few months:** Ibid., 33–35.

65 **Safar was given a medical discharge:** Ibid., 36–37.

65 **To keep them out:** Ibid., 39.

66 **Safar, exhausted and elated:** Ibid., 41.

66 **Safar was rebellious:** Ibid., 53.

67 **Vienna had become too small:** Ibid., 58.

68 **In class he was thrilled:** Ibid., 61.

68 **In Austria, anesthesia:** Ibid., 17.

68 **It was a brand-new field:** Ibid., 66.

68 **He'd met several women:** Ibid.

68 **He was a rascal:** Phone interview with Eva Safar, August 2020.

69 **This boy, the mischievous Peter:** Ibid.

69 **She knew right away:** Ibid.

69 **Safar too:** Safar, *Careers in Anesthesiology*, vol. 5, 46.

69 **She sensed, too:** Phone interview with Eva Safar, August 2020.

70 **"I'll go to the moon with you.":** Safar, *Careers in Anesthesiology*, vol. 5, 66.

CHAPTER ELEVEN

71 **David Lawrence's heart:** "Ex-Governor Stricken at Mosque Rally."

71 **Outside, politicians and reporters:** Ibid.

71 **When Lawrence first collapsed:** "Doctors Huddle over Lawrence," *Pittsburgh Post-Gazette*, November 5, 1966, 1.

71 **He was surprised:** Safar, *Careers in Anesthesiology,* vol. 5, 210.

71 **"clinically but not biologically" dead:** "Doctors Huddle over Lawrence."

72 **Safar was in charge:** Safar, *Careers in Anesthesiology*, vol. 5, 210.

72 **By this point:** "Doctors Huddle over Lawrence."

72 **He was now breathing:** Safar, *Careers in Anesthesiology*, vol. 5, 210.

73 **Safar stood back:** Ibid.

73 **This bout, the governor's second:** "Ex-Governor Stricken at Mosque Rally."

CHAPTER TWELVE

74 **Cyclopropane, halothane:** Safar, *Careers in Anesthesiology*, vol. 5, 129.

74 **Even when Safar wasn't working:** Phone interview with Eva Safar, August 2020; phone interview with Fran Mistrick, February 2019.

74 **It didn't sound as if:** *Careers in Anesthesiology*, vol. 5, 129.

74 **But people were still:** Ibid., 129–130.

75 **The key to it all:** Ibid., 129.

75 **To convince the rest of the world:** Ibid., 132.

75 **But everyone said no:** Ibid., 137.

76 **Eighty percent of the kids:** Ibid., 47–48; phone interview with Eva Safar, August 2020.

76 **It would be many years:** Safar, *Careers in Anesthesiology*, vol. 5, 48.

76 **Ignited by what later generations:** Phone interview with Eva Safar, August 2020; phone interview with Paul Safar, March 2019.

76 **His survival was a heavy weight:** Phone interview with Eva Safar, August 2020.

76 **But he was too determined:** Ibid.

77 **To capture it:** Safar, *Careers in Anesthesiology*, vol. 5, 132; *Respiratory Resuscitation Techniques: An Experimental Study*, Walter Reed Army Institute of Research Production, 1957.

77 **The sedatives, given first:** Safar, *Careers in Anesthesiology*, vol. 5, 134.

77 **Whatever the risks:** Ibid.

77 **It signaled their dedication:** Ibid.

77 **First, they would be treated:** Ibid., 132.

77 **Instead, the one method:** Ibid., 132–133.

78 **The first test was held:** Ibid., 132.

78 **Eva, too, stood among:** Phone interview with Eva Safar, August 2020.

78 **She would stop short:** Ibid.

78 **Elam was not entirely an ally:** Safar, *Careers in Anesthesiology*, vol. 5, 131.

79 **Chief Martin McMahon:** Ibid., 132.

79 **And if it were to happen now:** Phone interview with Eva Safar, August 2020.

80 **And what they showed:** Safar, *Careers in Anesthesiology*, vol. 5, 136.

80 **Unlike the victims:** Ibid., 135.

80 **With all the assurance of youth:** *Respiratory Resuscitation Techniques*.

81 **Elam was ecstatic:** "Mouth-to-Mouth Held Best Respiration Aid," *Los Angeles Times*, October 18, 1957, 18.

81 **"Either moved no air":** Ibid.

81 **"The old methods simply:** "For Reviving Near-Drowning Victims," *Miami Herald*, October 8, 1959, 65.

81 **A documentary, produced by the army:** *Respiratory Resuscitation Techniques*.

81 **And because there were sure:** Safar, *Careers in Anesthesiology*, vol. 5, 135–136.

81 **With the camera trained:** Ibid.

82 **But it was the arresting sight:** "Series Here to Demonstrate New Life-Saving Technique," *Daily Independent Journal* (San Rafael, CA), May 5, 1959, 3; "Mouth-to-Mouth Held Best Respiration Aid," *Los Angeles Times*, October 18, 1957, 18.

82 **Nearly a year to the day:** Safar, *Careers in Anesthesiology*, vol. 5, 137; "Mouth-to-Mouth Held Best Respiration Aid."

82 **"a bombshell in the US:** Safar, *Careers in Anesthesiology*, vol. 5, 137.

82 **The data and the documentary:** Ibid., 144.

83 **"overzealous rescuers":** Area Police Departments, Rescuers to Get Resuscitubes," *Sunday News* (Ridgewood, NJ), July 12, 1959, 8.

83 **In its August 1959 issue:** "New Method of Resuscitation Is Only 3,000 Years Old," *Asbury Park [NJ] Press*, August 23, 1959, 13.

83 **"Controversies, misunderstandings:** Safar, *Careers in Anesthesiology*, vol. 5, 140.

83 **Even as hand-wringing:** Ibid., 142.

CHAPTER THIRTEEN

84 **in the days after his collapse:** "Ex-Governor Shows Signs That End Near," *Pittsburgh Post-Gazette*, November 7, 1966, 1.

84 **"He's stubborn all over,":** Ibid.

84 **"I will not return to the campaign trail:** "Ex-Governor Stricken at Mosque Rally," 4.

84 **"stunned and grim-faced":** Ibid.

85 **Within hours of Lawrence's arrival:** "'No Chance,' Doctors say," *Pittsburgh Press*, November 6, 1966, 1; Safar, *Careers in Anesthesiology*, vol. 5, 210.

85 **Safar believed it was:** Ibid., 211.

85 **"slipped away":** "Lawrence 'Just Slipped Away,'" *Pittsburgh Press*, November 22, 1966, 4.

86 **He was committed:** Safar, *Careers in Anesthesiology*, vol. 5, 127.

86 **On the night of June 26:** Ibid., 197.

86 **Elizabeth had been born premature:** Phone interview with Eva Safar, August 2020.

86 **Asthma had plagued:** Safar, *Careers in Anesthesiology*, vol. 5, 13.

87 **He immediately took over:** Ibid., 197.

88 **And it had been even less time:** Ibid., 207.

89 **At four minutes to three:** "Big Ben Stops for 22 Minutes," *Pittsburgh Post-Gazette*, November 22, 1966, 1.

89 **"Lawrence detested maudlin:** "Eulogies Hail Public Servant Dave Lawrence," *Pittsburgh Press*, November 22, 1966, 1.

89 **State Supreme Court Justice:** Ibid.

89 **US Senator Joseph Clark:** Ibid.

89 **Farther afield, President Lyndon Johnson:** "Ex-Gov. Lawrence Dies After 17-Day Battle in Hospital," *Pittsburgh Post-Gazette*, November 22, 1966, 1.

89 **In the Pittsburgh offices:** Phone interview with Phil Hallen, June 2020.

90 **Hallen arrived:** Phone interview with Phil Hallen, February 2019.

90 **Realizing how outmatched:** Ibid.

90 **"Just stand back:** Bell, *The Ambulance*, 256.

90 **Not one to be lost:** Phone interview with Phil Hallen, February 2019.

91 **The poor state of ambulance care:** Phone interview with Phil Hallen, October 2019.

91 **"We're twenty-five years:** Ibid.

91 **In Pittsburgh, there were:** Phone interview with Phil Hallen, February 2019.

91 **The firehouses had:** Safar, *Careers in Anesthesiology*, vol. 5, 208.

91 **In the city's Black neighborhoods:** Phone interview with Phil Hallen, September 2018.

92 **And that's if they showed up:** Phone interview with John Moon, November 2018.

92 **Much like Safar:** Ibid.

92 **"I need to talk to Jim McCoy:** Phone interview with Phil Hallen, June 2020.

92 **Freedom House was the brainchild:** "The Life and Thoughts of James McCoy, Jr.," *Pittsburgh Press*, 11–13.

93 **Though it'd been:** Ibid.

93 **McCoy was no longer a young man:** Ibid.

93 **McCoy, a Black man:** Ibid.

94 **"A person does not get:** Ibid.

94 **And the plan he'd come to discuss:** Phone interview with Phil Hallen, June 2020.

94 **"little drops of water:** "The Life and Thoughts of James McCoy, Jr.," *Pittsburgh Press*, 11–13.

94 **He'd spent time in jail:** Trotter and Day, *Race and Renaissance*, 93.

95 **He was in:** Bell, *The Ambulance*, 261.

CHAPTER FIFTEEN

96 **"Go talk to Safar.":** Phone interview with Phil Hallen, June 2020.

96 **What he had, really:** Ibid.

96 **Safar did, of course:** Safar, *Careers in Anesthesiology*, vol. 5, 211.

97 **Safar told Hallen and McCoy:** Phone interview with Phil Hallen, September 2019.

97 **Instead, he wanted to train paramedics:** Ibid.; Safar, *Careers in Anesthesiology*, vol. 5, 211.

97 **Safar wanted to end:** Ibid., 210.

98 **Without realizing it:** Phone interview with Phil Hallen, September 2019.

98 **"I've been trying to figure:** Phone interview with Phil Hallen, June 2020.

98 **"So . . . we can certainly:** Ibid.

98 **"I'm trying to train people:** Ibid.

99 **"I want ordinary people,":** Ibid.

99 **"Oh, we have ordinary:** Ibid.

99 **"You've got the gas:** Ibid.

99 **For Hallen and McCoy:** Phone interview with Phil Hallen, September 2019.

99 **"unemployables,":** Phone interview with John Moon, September 2018; phone interview with Phil Hallen, October 2018; "'Unemployable' Provide Service," *Pittsburgh Post-Gazette*, April 9, 1969, 21.

100 **If they ever worried:** Safar, *Careers in Anesthesiology*, vol. 5, 211–212.

CHAPTER SIXTEEN

101 **The larger world:** Phone interview with Phil Hallen, June 2020.

101 **Aside from Safar and McCoy and Hallen:** Ibid.

101 **The first item:** Ibid.

102 **"How big?:** Ibid.

102 **"Okay," said Coleman:** Ibid.

103 **Envisioned in those early:** Bell, *The Ambulance*, 263.

103 **In those weekly:** James O. Page, *The Paramedics: An Illustrated History of Paramedics in Their First Decade in the U.S.A.* (Morristown, NJ: Backdraft Publications, 1979), 33.

103 **Support from the county:** Bell, *The Ambulance*, 262.

103 **Then there was the money:** Ibid., 263.

103 **By October:** Page, *The Paramedics*, 34.

103 **Before joining Freedom House:** "Gerald 'Jerry' Esposito, Founder of Ambulance Service Began with Station Wagon" (obituary), *Pittsburgh Post-Gazette*, May 31, 2003.

104 **This set off panic:** Page, *The Paramedics*, 34.

104 **Say what you want:** Bell, *The Ambulance*, 263.

104 **John Conley:** "Ambulance Service Comes to the Inner City," *Opportunity* (February 1971): 8.

104 **Thelma Lovette:** Phone interview with Phil Hallen, September 2019; "Thelma Lovette, Beloved Hill District Icon, Dies at 91," *New Pittsburgh Courier*, May 28, 2014.

104 **Together they roped in:** Bell, *The Ambulance*, 263.

CHAPTER SEVENTEEN

105 **In the morning:** "Emergency!" *Pittsburgh Magazine* (April 1977): 43.

105 **"I have one of those funny mind":** "Ex-Jobless Running to Rescue," *Pittsburgh Press*, November 17, 1968, 41.

105 **Dave Rayzer was married:** Ibid.

105 **Their ages ranged:** "Emergency!," 44; phone interview with John Moon, October 2018.

105 **Several had been:** "Six Juveniles, Youth Held in Stabbing of Marine," *Pittsburgh Post-Gazette*, December 28, 1963, 2; "The Forgotten Legacy of Freedom House," EMSWorld, April 29, 2019, www.emsworld.com/article/1222574/forgotten-legacy-freedom-house.

106 **"had little to look forward to":** "Ambulance Service Comes to the Inner City," *Opportunity* (February 1971): 8.

106 **Hallen was more anxious:** Phone interview with Phil Hallen, September 2019.

106 **The task before each:** "Emergency!," 44; Bell, *The Ambulance*, 265–267.

107 **"exponentially more training":** Ibid., 264.

107 **"Serial interrogations":** Ibid., 263.

107 **By the time the process:** Ibid.

107 **Tired and frustrated:** Benson, Esposito, Dirsch, et al., "Mobile Intensive Care by 'Unemployable' Blacks Trained as Emergency Medical Technicians (EMT's)," 408–421.

107 **It took a toll:** Ibid.

109 **Like that of other medical:** Phone interview with Phil Hallen, September 2019.

109 **Despite the patches:** Bell, *The Ambulance*, 266.

109 **The ER was another story:** Ibid., 267.

110 **"You have thirty seconds:** Phone interview with John Moon, November 2018.

111 **That the medics would:** Bell, *The Ambulance*, 265.

111 **He tried to convince other:** Phone interview with John Moon, September 2020.

112 **Reluctantly, Safar moved on:** Ibid.

112 **They rushed back to Pittsburgh:** "The Forgotten Legacy of Freedom House."

112 **$2.50 an hour:** Faulk Medical Fund archives, Heinz History Center, Pittsburgh.

113 **They understood the anger:** Phone interview with John Moon, November 2018.

113 **In this uniform:** Ibid.

CHAPTER EIGHTEEN

114 **This was the hotline:** "Ex-Jobless Rushing to Rescue," *Pittsburgh Press*, November 17, 1968, 41.

114 **The automatic doors:** Ibid.

114 **His partner, Morant:** Ibid.

115 **Another Oakland overdose:** Ibid.

116 **Five months before, on July 15:** Bell, *The Ambulance*, 267.

116 **Freedom House had coasted:** Ibid., 268–269; phone interview with Phil Hallen, February 2019; "Emergency!," 46.

116 **He got money:** phone interview with Phil Hallen, February 2019; "Ex-Jobless Running to Rescue"; Bell, *The Ambulance*, 269.

116 **In the first year alone:** "Ambulance Score," *Pittsburgh Press*, January 11, 1970, 21.

117 **When not on calls:** "'Super' Ambulances Make Debut Here," *Pittsburgh Press*, April 8, 1969, 12.

117 **By the spring of 1969:** Ibid.

117 **Safar was a pioneer:** Safar, *Careers in Anesthesiology*, vol. 5, 152; "Peter Safar, Cardiopulmonary Resuscitation," Lemelson-MIT, lemelson.mit.edu/resources/peter-safar, accessed March 4, 2022.

117 **They were modified and equipped:** Phone interview with Phil Hallen, February 2019.

117 **A sense of ownership:** Phone interview with John Moon, May 2019.

118 **The base station at Presby:** Phone interview with John Moon, February 2020.

118 **Player, gambler, ladies' man:** Phone interview with Bill Raynovich, October 2020.

118 **He would tell people:** Diary/notes from the Papers of Nancy L. Caroline, 1905–2007, Schlesinger Library, Radcliffe Institute, Harvard University.

118 **Trouble with a new girl:** Phone interview with John Moon, February 2020.

118 **There was Curtis Scott:** Phone interview with Bill Raynovich, October 2020.

118 **"The time for action:** Emergency!," 46.

119 **"It was the biggest thing,":** "Pioneer Medics to Gather Again," *Pittsburgh Post-Gazette*, November 7, 1997, 25.

119 **On calls, kids gathered:** "Ex-Jobless Rushing to Rescue."

119 **Dave Thomas turned twenty-one:** "Ambulance Service Comes to the Inner City," *Opportunity* (February 1971): 8.

119 **for far too long, Black men:** Phone interview with John Moon, December 2018.

119 **"It makes me . . . proud":** "Ex-Jobless Rushing to Rescue."

CHAPTER NINETEEN

120 **Even though they were now funded:** "Emergency!," 46.

120 **They were reliant on donations:** "City Puts Brakes to Blacks' Ambulance Runs," *Pittsburgh Press*, January 11, 1970, 21.

120 **Mitch Brown grew up:** "A Departing Mitch Brown Looks Back," *University Times*, January 24, 1980, 2.

120 **But Mitch was determined:** Ibid.

121 **One day in August:** Mitch Brown, remarks during webinar hosted by the University of Pittsburgh Graduate School of Public Health, September 2020.

121 **He never again:** Ibid.

121 **That fall he left:** "A Departing Mitch Brown Looks Back."

122 **"I'm better than anybody:** Mitch Brown, remarks during webinar.

122 **Brown might've been cocky:** Phone interview with John Moon, February 2021.

122 **"We're going to make you into:** "A Departing Mitch Brown Looks Back."

122 **"you can't forget:** Ibid.

122 **Mitch was outspoken:** Mitch Brown, remarks during webinar.

123 **"We don't need any:** Ibid.

123 **"We have to do this:** Ibid.

123 **"In that case:** Ibid.

123 **The guy's name has been lost:** Phone interview with Bill Raynovich, October 2020.

123 **At that very moment:** Ibid.

124 **Raynovich crawled in:** Ibid.

124 **After high school:** Ibid.

125 **When Raynovich arrived:** Ibid.

126 **For his new coworkers:** Phone interview with John Moon, August 2020; phone interview with Darnella Wilson, August 2020.

126 **Many were skeptical:** Phone interview with John Moon, August 2020.

127 **If Raynovich was being sized up:** Phone interview with Bill Raynovich, October 2020.

CHAPTER TWENTY

128 **By 1972:** "Telemetry Keeps Doctor, Emergency Unit in Touch," *Pittsburgh Press*, July 25, 1972, 7.

128 **The world began to take note:** Ibid.

128 **Since Safar's specially designed ambulances:** From the Papers of Nancy L. Caroline, 1905–2007, Schlesinger Library, Radcliffe Institute, Harvard University.

128 **Back in the late '50s:** Phone interview with Eva Safar, August 2020; Safar, *Careers in Anesthesiology*, vol. 5, 138.

128 **Freedom House also reintroduced:** Bell, *The Ambulance*, 276

129 **In 1967, Miami's Dr. Eugene Nagel:** Ibid., 284.

129 **Take the city's nurses:** "Student Nurses Hit Road," *Pittsburgh Press*, January 30, 1972, 81.

129 **"fabulous! They are so cool!":** Ibid.

129 **Sometimes they slept:** Phone interview with John Moon, March 2021.

130 **Mitch said no:** Mitch Brown, remarks during webinar.

130 **"that there is no evidence:** Typed job description of Freedom House Medical Director, from the Papers of Nancy L. Caroline.

130 **At the time, Pittsburgh was:** Mitch Brown, remarks during webinar.

130 **Over a two-month period in 1972:** "Telemetry Keeps Doctor, Emergency Units in Touch."

131 **Police and fire departments:** Safar, *Careers in Anesthesiology*, vol. 5, 208.

131 **A Freedom House crew:** "Telemetry Keeps Doctor, Emergency Units in Touch."

131 **It cost much less:** Ibid.

CHAPTER TWENTY-ONE

134 **On his very first shift:** Phone interview with John Moon, May 2019.

134 **Months back, when he first barged:** Ibid.

135 **He was still working:** Phone interview with John Moon, November 2018.

135 **It was early evening:** Phone interview with John Moon, February 2021.

136 **There was only fear:** Ibid.

136 **It was the city's first:** "On This Day," WPXI News, April 15, 2020, www.wpxi.com/archive/this-day-april-15-1940-construction-bedford-dwellings-is-completed/UJZDW2YI7ZHBDHEOEKHEO3TF5Y.

136 **Now mothers chased:** "Bedford Dwellings," *Pittsburgh Post-Gazette*, May 30, 2014.

137 **John wasn't really there:** Phone interview with John Moon, February 2021.

137 **"Burns are third-degree.":** Ibid.

138 **"We gotta get this off.":** Ibid.

139 **Holland was strict:** Ibid.

140 **George McCary joined:** Phone interview with George McCary, March 2019.

140 **All he wanted:** Ibid.

140 **"You got to go,":** Brett Williams, "Freedom House: A Rich History and a Continuing Legacy: An Interview with George McCary," *Australasian Journal of Paramedicine* 12, no. 3 (2015).

140 **One of George's cousins:** Ibid.

140 **George saw himself:** Phone interview with George McCary, March 2019.

140 **"I'm not doing this for me,":** Williams, "Freedom House."

140 **George fell in love with it:** Phone interview with George McCary, March 2019.

141 **By his own estimation:** Ibid.

141 **John so serious:** Phone interview with John Moon, May 2021.

141 **"But I came out smelling:** Phone interview with George McCary, March 2019.

141 **"Hey man!:** Phone interview with John Moon, May 2021.

142 **"There you go.":** Ibid.

143 **The shell he'd retreated into:** Ibid.

CHAPTER TWENTY-TWO

144 **In the early hours:** "Homewood Killing Laid to Drug Row," *Pittsburgh Post-Gazette*, January 18, 1972, 10.

144 **Harrington later said:** "New Yorker Found Guilty of Killing City Man," *Pittsburgh Press*, September 26, 1972, 5.

144 **"bullet-ridden":** Ibid.

144 **His murderer was arrested:** Ibid.

145 **Two years earlier, Carl Staten:** "Mate Slain, Wife Charged," *Pittsburgh Post-Gazette*, October 17, 1970, 16.

145 **The medics seemed almost relieved:** Phone interview with John Moon, February 2021.

145 **"We had all the momentum:** Hunter S. Thompson, *Fear and Loathing in Las Vegas: A Savage Journey to the Heart of the American Dream* (New York: Warner Books, 1982).

146 **what he would call the "silent majority,":** "Who Speaks for the Majority," *New York Times*, November 2, 2011.

146 **Claiming to speak for the "forgotten Americans:** Ibid.

146 **With boos and jeers:** "Pittsburgh Mayor, at Public Inauguration, Vows a Housecleaning," *New York Times*, January 6, 1970.

147 **In a Kennedy-esque gesture:** Ibid.

147 **The protesters were there:** Ibid.

147 **Born on June 24:** Peter F. Flaherty Papers, 1964–1995, Archives & Special Collections, University of Pittsburgh Library System.

147 **It was there that he caught:** "Peter Flaherty Dies at 80," *Pittsburgh Post-Gazette*, April 19, 2005, https://www.post-gazette.com/news/obituaries/2005/04/19/Obituary-Pete-Flaherty-dies-at-80/stories/200504190204.

147 **It was a decision:** Ibid.

147 **"Nobody's Boy,":** Ibid.

147 **a whole new style of politics:** Ibid.

148 **Right out of the gate:** Ibid.

CHAPTER TWENTY-THREE

149 **Just after his inauguration:** "City Puts Brakes to Blacks' Ambulance Runs," *Pittsburgh Press*, January 11, 1970, 21.

149 **"The service is excellent,":** Ibid.

149 **To everyone involved:** Phone interview with John Moon, November 2018.

149 **In the past year alone:** "Ambulance Score," *Pittsburgh Press*, January 11, 1970, 21.

149 **When that man walked out:** Phone interview with John Moon, November 2018.

150 **So Safar and Hallen:** Bell, *The Ambulance*, 270.

150 **In 1972, Safar began rattling:** Ibid., 271.

150 **"We already have:** "Flaherty Unmoved on Future Aid for Freedom House," *Pittsburgh Post-Gazette*, June 22, 1974, 11.

150 **This *good* service:** "Going to Proper Hospital Vital," *Pittsburgh Press*, July 26, 1972, 25; "Lives Hinge on Better Emergency Care, Wecht Says," *Pittsburgh Press*, May 15, 1973, 21.

151 **Aside from being old:** "Too Often, Distress Call Brings Ride to Eternity," *Pittsburgh Press*, July 23, 1972, 39.

151 **"I get about thirty:** "Lives Hinge on Better Emergency Care."

151 **"If they're well-dressed:** Ibid.

151 **"amateurly run":** "Emergency Situation," *Pittsburgh Post-Gazette*, July 15, 1972, 4.

151 **One afternoon, Benson said:** "Too Often, Distress Call Brings Ride to Eternity."

151 **He fired off a passionate:** From the Papers of Nancy L. Caroline, 1905–2007, Schlesinger Library, Radcliffe Institute, Harvard University.

152 **Safar's letter was signed:** Ibid.

152 **His combative tone:** "Ex-Commissioner William Hunt Is Dead at 76," *Pittsburgh Post-Gazette*, July 21, 1990, 8.

152 **"an obstructionist,":** Ibid.

152 **"defaming and insulting":** "Hunt, Pitt Doctor Trade Views in City Ambulance Service Battle," *Pittsburgh Press*, May 6, 1973, 22.

152 **"the police have passed even:** Ibid.

153 **"very difficult and controversial:** Ibid.; Bell, *The Ambulance*, 270.

153 **"There are differences of opinion:** "Hunt, Pitt Doctor Trade Views in City Ambulance Service Battle."

153 **"a very difficult, complex question.":** "Flaherty Unmoved on Future Aid for Freedom House."

153 **Legitimate efforts had been made:** "Too Often, Distress Call Brings Ride to Eternity."

153 **Miami started a paramedic program:** Bell, *The Ambulance*, 284–285.

153 **Los Angeles started its:** Ibid., 287.

153 **Jacksonville's public safety director:** "Her Heart Failed 3 Times, But Rescue Squad Didn't," *Pittsburgh Press*, May 13, 1973, 41.

153 **Since launching their own paramedic:** Ibid.

153 **The call involved a fifty-year-old:** Ibid.

154 **"I was clinically dead three times,":** Ibid.

154 **San Francisco's repatriated:** "Cities Across U.S. Get Advanced Emergency Services on the Road," *Pittsburgh Press*, May 4, 1973, 25.

154 **LA—soon to be lionized:** Page, *The Paramedics*, 18.

154 **"equally competent medical authorities":** Bell, *The Ambulance*, 270.

154 **"The county is not:** "District Lets Medical Service Funds Slip Away," *Pittsburgh Press*, July 27, 1972, 31.

155 **"legal concerns":** "Continuation of Ambulance Up to Board," *Pittsburgh Press*, June 22, 1974, 2.

155 **Kane Hospital:** "District Lets Medical Service Funds Slip Away."

155 **Flaherty could only smile:** "Continuation of Ambulance Up to Board."

155 **By 1972, as the mayor dragged:** "Cities Across U.S. Get Advanced Emergency Services on the Road."

155 **But rather than collect:** "Her Heart Failed 3 Times, But Rescue Squad Didn't."

155 **There was also private:** "Stone Prods Pete to Get Ambulances," *Pittsburgh Press*, June 16, 1974, 19.

155 **"I want to make sure:** Ibid.

155 **Without asking for a dime:** "Just How Much Is a Life Worth?" *Pittsburgh Press*, May 16, 1973, 25.

156 **Freedom House Board member:** Faulk Medical Fund archives, Heinz History Center, Pittsburgh; "NAACP Protests End to Ambulance Service," *Pittsburgh Post-Gazette*, June 15, 1974, 11.

156 **Citizen's groups in:** "Let Freedom House Serve the Whole City," *Pittsburgh Post-Gazette*, June 22, 1974.

156 **"It doesn't make sense:** Bell, *The Ambulance*, 272.

157 **Richard Dixon:** "Freedom House Ambulance Funding Challenged," *Pittsburgh Press*, March 5, 1974, 9.

157 **"five or six years ago,":** Ibid.

157 **Still, his requests to expand:** "Continuation of Ambulance Up to Board."

157 **wasn't a life worth:** "Just How Much Is a Life Worth?"

CHAPTER TWENTY-FOUR

158 **Down at the base station:** Phone interview with John Moon, January 2019.

158 **Nobody actually believed:** Bell, *The Ambulance*, 272.

158 **It hadn't escaped John's attention:** Phone interview with John Moon, January 2019.

158 **The mayor had begun his tenure:** "Peter Flaherty Dies at 80."

158 **and further antagonized the city's cops:** "Flaherty to Delay Police Transfers, Arbitration OK'd," Pittsburgh Post-Gazette, April 23, 1970, 1.

158 **Handing ambulance operations:** Bell, *The Ambulance*, 270.

159 **his politics had been steadily drifting right:** "Flaherty Antiblack, Irvis Laments," *Pittsburgh Post-Gazette*, March 26, 1975, 17.

159 **He came out against school busing:** Ibid.

159 **"The real tragedy:** Ibid.

159 **"It just ain't fashionable:** "Hill House Geared to Meet Almost Anyone's Needs," *Pittsburgh Post-Gazette*, March 26, 1975, 17.

159 **Phil Hallen tended to agree:** Phone interview with Phil Hallen, September 2019.

159 **"outright racist":** Ibid.

160 **The guys at Freedom House:** Phone interview with John Moon, November 2018; phone interview with Bill Raynovich, October 2020.

160 **"This is stupid.":** Phone interview with John Moon, January 2021.

161 **"reckless driving of ambulances,":** "Ambulance Speed Rapped by Hunt," *Pittsburgh Post-Gazette*, April 6, 1972, 19.

161 **Hunt was helpful enough:** Ibid.

161 **The ban, of course:** "Hunt Urges Ambulance Speed Curbs," *Pittsburgh Press*, April 5, 1972, 11.

161 **The vans had heat:** Phone interview with John Moon, March 2020.

161 **The door fell off Unit 2:** "Report to the FHE Board," June 1975, from the Papers of Nancy L. Caroline, 1905–2007, Schlesinger Library, Radcliffe Institute, Harvard University.

162 **It felt to him:** Phone interview with John Moon, November 2018.

162 **George pointed out:** Phone interview with John Moon, February 2019.

162 **But George just walked in:** Ibid.; Brett Williams, "Freedom House: A Rich History and a Continuing Legacy: An Interview with George McCary," *Australasian Journal of Paramedicine* 12, no. 3 (2015).

163 **But then it's possible, too:** Phone interview with John Moon, February 2019; Bell, *The Ambulance*, 275.

163 **"Do you really have to do this?":** Phone interview with John Moon, February 2019.

164 **"What the hell are you doing?":** Ibid.

164 **"If he dies:** Ibid.

164 **It was uglier:** Ibid.

164 **"Without care you could die.":** Ibid.

165 **It happened again:** Ibid.

165 **"spite selling":** "Black Just Wanted Home, White Family Sold Its Out of Fear," *Pittsburgh Post-Gazette*, August 8, 1973, 4.

165 **When John leapt:** Phone interview with John Moon, May 2020.

166 **Not even fifteen minutes:** Ibid.

166 **Just the year before:** "Feb. 17, 1972: Beetle Outruns Model T," *Wired*, February 17, 2010.

166 **Safar had taught his medics:** Phone interview with John Moon, May 2020.

166 **"No! No, no, no, no, no!":** Ibid.

167 **"a person with a damaged:** "Lives Hinge on Better Emergency Care, Wecht Says," *Pittsburgh Press*, May 15, 1973, 21.

167 **"You can't do that!:** Phone interview with John Moon, May 2020.

167 **"Get the fuck out of here!":** Ibid.

167 **"You want me to put your ass in jail?":** Ibid.

168 **It was frustrating and embarrassing:** Ibid.

168 **All the way back in 1967:** Bell, *The Ambulance*, 262.

168 **It was a clash of styles:** Phone interview with John Moon, November 2018; phone interview with George McCary, March 2019; "Freedom House Aides' Hopes Fading," *Pittsburgh Post-Gazette*, June 20, 1974, 13.

168 **The cops were focused on:** Phone interview with John Moon, November 2018; phone interview with George McCary, March 2019.

168 **"When Freedom House goes:** "Freedom House Aides' Hopes Fading."

168 **The other medics:** Phone interview with John Moon, May 2020.

168 **"Yeah,":** "Freedom House Aides' Hopes Fading."

169 **"The police are trained to be hard:** Ibid.

169 **August 1968:** Trotter and Day, *Race and Renaissance*, 107.

169 **April 1970:** "Flaherty to Delay Police Transfers, Arbitration OK'd."

169 **Fall 1972:** Trotter and Day, *Race and Renaissance*, 127.

169 **That members of the Pittsburgh police:** Ibid.

169 **"abuse anyone who dared:** Ibid., 125.

169 **"too ingrained with racism:** Ibid., 127.

169 **a white cop running for office:** "Black Detective Seeks Redress," *Pittsburgh Post-Gazette*, June 20, 1974, 13.

170 **The people at the top:** Phone interview with John Moon, May 2020.

170 **To hell with everyone else:** Ibid.

CHAPTER TWENTY-FIVE

172 **A crisp fall day:** "Medical Rescue Plan Keeps Pitt Fan Alive," *Pittsburgh Press*, September 28, 1975, 22.

173 **A twenty-five-year-old man:** "Man Threatens Police in Oakland Standoff," *Pittsburgh Post-Gazette*, July 20, 1974, 3.

173 **an eighty-one-year-old woman:** "Guard Injured Catching Child From 3 Stories," *Pittsburgh Post-Gazette*, October 24, 1974, 1.

174 **Inside the hushed security:** "Ambulance Crew Wins Commendation," *Pittsburgh Press*, February 18, 1975.

174 **Medics were dragged back:** Phone interview with John Moon, May 2019.

CHAPTER TWENTY-SIX

176 **Nancy Caroline was working:** "Emergency!," 45.

176 **"Dr. Safar has a:** Ibid.

177 **"It can be arranged,":** Diary/notes from the Papers of Nancy L. Caroline, 1905–2007.

177 **"Because," Edelstein cut in:** Ibid.

177 **"Scan this material:** Ibid.

178 **In such a climate:** "City Plans to Buy 5 Heart Ambulances," *Pittsburgh Press*, March 11, 1974, 1; "Pete Lauded on Buying Plan," *Pittsburgh Press*, March 12, 1974, 7.

178 **the city council openly endorsed:** "Emergency Ambulance Setup OK'd," *Pittsburgh Post-Gazette*, March 12, 1974, 13.

178 **He refused:** "Pete Ambulances Over a Hurdle," *Pittsburgh Press*, March 14, 1974, 54; "New Ambulance Plan," *Pittsburgh Press*, March 14, 1974, 32.

178 **In his 1974 budget proposal:** "New Ambulance Plan."

178 **Frustrated, the council acted:** Ibid.

178 **Though Flaherty refused to sign:** Ibid.

178 **But nobody knew:** Ibid.

178 **five specialized ambulances:** "Emergency Ambulance Setup OK'd."

179 **Colville concluded:** Ibid.

179 **"would be a mistake,":** "Pete Lauded on Buying Plan."

179 **"Whether his present aspirations:** Ibid.

179 **"That the Mayor did not:** Ibid.

179 **Flaherty wanted only:** Ibid.; "City Plans to Buy 5 Heart Ambulances."

179 **That they were already better:** "Keep Freedom House," *Pittsburgh Post-Gazette*, June 19, 1974, 6.

179 **Opponents of this plan:** Ibid.

179 **Press conferences were:** "NAACP Protests End to Ambulance Service," *Pittsburgh Post-Gazette*, June 15, 1974, 11.

179 **They came from all over:** "Freedom House Support Mounting," *Pittsburgh Press*, June 15, 1974, 2.

180 **"Freedom House would be replaced:** "NAACP Protests End to Ambulance Service."

180 **"It is foolish and insulting:** "Freedom House Support Mounting."

180 **the *Post-Gazette* noted:** "Keep Freedom House."

180 **he viewed as background noise:** Phone interview with John Moon, November 2018.

180 **His son, John, was five:** Phone interview with John Moon, November 2021.

180 **He arrived in the middle of the night:** Ibid.

181 **But not everyone was able:** "Freedom House Aides' Hopes Fading," *Pittsburgh Post-Gazette*, June 20, 1974, 13.

181 **"If a guy has OD'd:** Ibid.

181 **"We have expert:** "Freedom House Support Mounting."

181 **"How would you like:** Bell, *The Ambulance*, 275.

181 **Ordinary citizens also came forward:** "Freedom House Didn't Fail Us," *Pittsburgh Post-Gazette*, June 22, 1974.

181 **"Why should the police:** "Let Freedom House Serve the Whole City," *Pittsburgh Post-Gazette*, June 22, 1974, op-ed.

181 **budget constraints had kept:** "'Happy Medium Ambulance Service,'" *Pittsburgh Post-Gazette*, July 3, 1974, 6.

182 **Fact is, Freedom House was on the brink:** "Freedom House Aides' Hopes Fading"; "Continuation of Ambulance up to Board," *Pittsburgh*

Press, June 22, 1974, 2; "Flaherty Unmoved on Future Aid for Freedom House," *Pittsburgh Post-Gazette*, June 22, 1974, 11.

182 **When he heard this news:** "Flaherty Unmoved on Future Aid for Freedom House."

182 **Police Superintendent Colville:** "Service Extended by Freedom House," *Pittsburgh Press*, June 18, 1974, 6.

182 **"It would be the height of irony:** "Hope Not Dead for Freedom House," *Pittsburgh Press*, June 14, 1974, 24.

182 **"a pattern of ripoff:** "NAACP Protests End to Ambulance Service."

182 **He switched tactics:** "Flaherty Unmoved on Future Aid for Freedom House."

183 **On July 3:** "2 Brothers, 3rd Suspect Sought," *Pittsburgh Press*, July 3, 1974, 1.

183 **"bad actors":** Ibid.

183 **One night, officers:** "2 Northside Men Allege Mistreatment by Police," *Pittsburgh Post-Gazette*, August 7, 1974, 1.

183 **"I'll kill the:** Ibid.

183 **On another occasion:** "Police Defend Tactics in Officer Killer Hunt," *Pittsburgh Post-Gazette*, July 10, 1974, 1.

183 **"Things are tense:** "Strain of Manhunt Shows, Cops Admit," *Pittsburgh Press*, July 9, 1974, 2.

183 **State Attorney General:** "Packel Pushes Brutality Probe," *Pittsburgh Press*, July 12, 1974, 4.

184 **The training, initially set:** "Pete Ripped in Ambulance Stall," *Pittsburgh Press*, June 9, 1974, 8; "City to Ask Bids on Ambulance Super-Fleet," *Pittsburgh Press*, October 13, 1974, 2.

184 **They were now due to arrive in January:** Ibid.

184 **"If this was mostly:** "Freedom House Aides' Hopes Fading."

184 **Flaherty was forced to relent:** "Freedom House Gets Funds for 75," *Pittsburgh Post-Gazette*, September 24, 1974, 13.

CHAPTER TWENTY-SEVEN

185 **This was the last straw:** "Emergency!," 84.

185 **High on the group's list:** Ibid.

186 **The organization had become disorganized:** Ibid.

186 **Though he created:** Safar, *Careers in Anesthesiology*, vol. 5, 213, 234.

186 **Included in all this:** Ibid., 234.

186 **He had nobody:** Diary/notes from the Papers of Nancy Caroline, 1905–2007.

187 **Those he'd managed to snare:** Safar, *Careers in Anesthesiology*, vol. 5, 234.

CHAPTER TWENTY-EIGHT

188 **Nancy was always of two minds:** Diary/notes from the Papers of Nancy L. Caroline, 1905–2007.

188 **relationships with impossible men:** Ibid.

188 **Nancy Caroline was born:** Introduction to the Papers of Nancy L. Caroline.

188 **She flushed the toilet:** Diary/notes from the Papers of Nancy L. Caroline.

189 **Maybe it was better:** Ibid.

189 **So after she graduated:** Phone interview with Peter Caroline, February 2019.

189 **"I try to care for:** Pamphlet on Case Western from the Papers of Nancy L. Caroline.

190 **She nearly dropped out:** Phone interview with Peter Caroline, February 2019.

190 **"a badge of independence":** Letter to Nancy from her uncle, David Stearns, from the Papers of Nancy L. Caroline.

190 **She graduated in 1971:** Diary/notes from the Papers of Nancy L. Caroline.

190 **When she hit Pittsburgh:** Ibid.

190 **Her cousin Audrey:** Phone interview with Audrey Schoenweld, September 2020.

190 **Nancy smoked a lot:** "Terrorists! Med-Emergency!" *Jewish Chronicle of Pittsburgh*, April 26, 1979, 8.

190 **It was August, she'd barely:** Diary/notes from the Papers of Nancy L. Caroline.

190 **And now, three months later:** "Emergency!," 45.

191 **She was intrigued:** Diary/notes from the Papers of Nancy L. Caroline.

191 **Nancy was a born contrarian:** Phone interview with Peter Caroline, February 2019.

191 **The next day, she responded:** Letter from Nancy Caroline to Peter Safar, November 1974, from the Papers of Nancy L. Caroline.

191 **Nancy at first said no:** Ibid.

192 **Pitt University health system was considered:** Phone interview with Eva Safar, August 2020; Safar, *Careers in Anesthesiology*, vol. 5, 161–165.

192 **He was so excited:** Phone interview with Paul Safar, March 2019; Safar, *Careers in Anesthesiology*, vol. 5, 160.

192 **He never even inquired:** Safar, *Careers in Anesthesiology*, vol. 5, 167.

192 **For most doctors:** Ibid., 175.

192 **So Safar turned his energy:** Ibid., 176–177.

192 **He assured her:** Letter from Nancy Caroline to Peter Safar, November 1974.

193 **Safar was triumphant:** Letter from Peter Safar to Nancy Caroline, December 1974, from the Papers of Nancy L. Caroline.

193 **"not as bad as it seems":** "Emergency!"

CHAPTER TWENTY-NINE

194 **"Now look, fellas:** Diary/notes from the Papers of Nancy L. Caroline, 1905–2007.

194 **what choice did he have:** Phone interview with John Moon, December 2020.

195 **if she was good enough for:** Ibid.

195 **Across town, Nancy sat:** Diary/notes from the Papers of Nancy L. Caroline.

195 **Very quickly Nancy's:** Ibid.

195 **Heightened stakes were added:** Nancy Caroline, draft of "Emergency Care in the Streets," from the Papers of Nancy L. Caroline.

195 **In Miami she felt:** Diary/notes from the Papers of Nancy L. Caroline.

196 **"We try not to bring:** Ibid.

196 **Manny, a forty-four-year-old:** Obituary for Manuel Soto Curiel, *Kansas City Star*, March 16, 1975, 8.

196 **Things got serious:** Diary/notes from the Papers of Nancy L. Caroline.

196 **She signed her letters:** Note from Nancy Caroline to Manuel Curiel, from the Papers of Nancy L. Caroline.

196 **Manny drank:** Letter from Nancy Caroline to Manuel Curiel, July 1974, from the Papers of Nancy L. Caroline; letter to Dr. Jonathan Gill from Nancy Caroline, January 1974, from the Papers of Nancy L. Caroline.

197 **"Rain the interminable,":** Diary/notes from the Papers of Nancy L. Caroline.

197 **"waiting for meaning:** Ibid.

198 **Nancy's first memorable:** Diary/notes from the Papers of Nancy L. Caroline, 1905–2007.

198 **There was no uniformity:** "Emergency!," 45.

199 **"maximally obnoxious.":** Ibid.

199 **"Orwellian reign of terror.":** Ibid.

199 **John's first indication:** Phone interview with John Moon, December 2018.

200 **She instituted weekly debriefings:** "Emergency!"

200 **The first time John was interrogated:** Phone interview with John Moon, December 2018.

200 **Attendance dwindled so much:** "Emergency!"

200 **She wanted her voice in their heads:** Ibid.

201 **A suicide, a premature birth:** Diary/notes from the Papers of Nancy L. Caroline.

201 **The first time she trailed John:** Phone interview with John Moon, December 2018.

201 **"We are a red light:** Diary/notes from the Papers of Nancy L. Caroline.

201 **"the squalor and misery:** Ibid.

201 **Today I careened:** Ibid.

202 **She put a cot in the bunk room:** Phone interview with John Moon, December 2018; phone interview with Bill Raynovich, October 2020.

202 **with paramedics Davis and McDoodle:** Diary/notes from the Papers of Nancy L. Caroline.

202 **another was the time Nancy and Ragin:** Ibid.

202 **Safar pulled her aside one morning:** Ibid.

203 **they started to complain:** Letter from Nancy Caroline to Peter Safar, February 1975, from the Papers of Nancy L. Caroline.

203 **(Safar questioning her time:** Letter from Peter Safar to Nancy Caroline, February 1975, from the Papers of Nancy L. Caroline.

203 **where they had no idea of her troubles:** Phone interview with John Moon, December 2018; phone interview with Bill Raynovich, October 2020.

203 **a grudging respect from even the most:** Phone interview with John Moon, December 2018; diary/notes from the Papers of Nancy L. Caroline.

203 **Walt Brown, whose explosive laugh:** Diary/notes from the Papers of Nancy L. Caroline.

203 **Too many cigarettes:** Ibid.

204 **"at the edge of madness,":** Ibid.

204 **an eight-year-old boy knocked senseless:** Ibid.

204 **basement of the ALCOA building:** Ibid.

204 **"Yours was the filet of sole, wasn't it?":** "Medical Care in the Streets," *Journal of the American Medical Association* (January 1977): 43.

204 **going down in a sewer with George:** Diary/notes from the Papers of Nancy L. Caroline.

204 **Nancy wasn't like Safar's other:** Phone interview with John Moon, December 2018.

204 **"place is legit,":** Diary/notes from the Papers of Nancy L. Caroline.

205 **Since coming to Pittsburgh:** Letter from Nancy Caroline to Peter Safar, May 1975, from the Papers of Nancy L. Caroline.

CHAPTER THIRTY-ONE

206 **The class was Safar's idea:** Phone interview with John Moon, February 2021.

206 **Now it was about survival:** Ibid.

206 **Every day, from eight:** Ibid.

207 **They pushed back:** Ibid.

207 **"pixie":** "Terrorists! Med-Emergency!" *Jewish Chronicle of Pittsburgh*, April 26, 1979, 8; "Dying in Academe," *New Physician* (November 1972): 656.

207 **"If you don't learn to speak like they do,":** Phone interview with John Moon, February 2021.

207 **She'd pressure Safar:** Ibid.

208 **He was marveling:** Ibid.

208 **He felt ten feet tall:** Ibid.

208 **One day John walked into:** Ibid.

208 **To John, Safar was a suggestion:** Ibid.

209 **John froze:** Ibid.

210 **Safar was elated:** Ibid.

CHAPTER THIRTY-TWO

212 **In March, Nancy was asked:** Diary/notes from the Papers of Nancy L. Caroline, 1905–2007.

212 **The following month:** "Report to the FHE Board," June 1975, from the Papers of Nancy L. Caroline.

212 **The physician in charge of:** Letter from Peter Haupert to Nancy Caroline, May 1975, from the Papers of Nancy L. Caroline.

212 **Nancy sensed the gathering:** Diary/notes from the Papers of Nancy L. Caroline.

213 **"a moment of impudent enthusiasm,":** Ibid.

213 **Nancy drew up a detailed:** "Disaster Drill" script, from the Papers of Nancy L. Caroline.

213 **For providers used to:** Phone interview with John Moon, February 2019.

214 **"half a dozen people:** Diary/notes from the Papers of Nancy L. Caroline.

214 **Nancy began to think:** Ibid.

214 **"I'm giving you the job:** Ibid.

214 **"threatened, bullied:** Ibid.

215 **She spoke to the cops:** Letter from Nancy Caroline to Peter Safar, March 1975, from the Papers of Nancy L. Caroline.

215 **Colville told Dr. Caroline:** Ibid.

215 **Insomuch as there can be:** Diary/notes from the Papers of Nancy L. Caroline.

216 **The mood in the base station:** Phone interview with John Moon, March 2021.

216 **One day Nancy blew through the door:** Ibid.

CHAPTER THIRTY-THREE

217 **She was up in the passenger seat:** Diary/notes from the Papers of Nancy L. Caroline, 1905–2007.

217 **Trying but failing:** Ibid.

218 **The day Nancy stormed:** Phone interview with John Moon, March 2021.

218 **And not just any voice but:** Ibid.

218 **Somehow Nancy had gotten:** Ibid.

218 **In short order:** Ibid.; diary/notes from the Papers of Nancy L. Caroline.

218 **They were overstepping:** Phone interview with John Moon, November 2018.

218 **a call for a man cut up:** Diary/notes from the Papers of Nancy L. Caroline.

219 **She rolled her eyes:** Ibid.

219 **Whatever funk she sank into:** Ibid.; phone interview with Darnella Wilson, August 2020.

219 **One night, about three thirty:** Diary/notes from the Papers of Nancy L. Caroline.

220 **"Happened to be in the neighborhood.":** Ibid.

220 **He'd shoot up a big:** Phone interview with John Moon, November 2018.

220 **Late one afternoon the scanner:** Phone interview with John Moon, February 2019; diary/notes from the Papers of Nancy L. Caroline.

223 **"We've got to work:** Diary/notes from the Papers of Nancy L. Caroline.

CHAPTER THIRTY-FOUR

224 **On the morning of the disaster:** Diary/notes from the Papers of Nancy L. Caroline, 1905–2007; "District Ambulance Plan Called Model for Country," *Pittsburgh Press*, May 9, 1975, 2.

224 **Relief was most definitely not:** Diary/notes from the Papers of Nancy L. Caroline.

224 **Feedback squealed through:** Ibid.

225 **"This is a multi-casualty disaster:** "Disaster Drill" script, from the Papers of Nancy L. Caroline.

225 **"If this happens:** Ibid.

225 **John threw his truck:** Phone interview with John Moon, February 2019.

225 **Nancy's stomach was in knots:** Diary/notes from the Papers of Nancy L. Caroline.

225 ***Yeah, I'm gonna show*:** Phone interview with John Moon, February 2019.

226 **When the last ambulance pulled away:** Diary/notes from the Papers of Nancy L. Caroline.

226 **To John, it was no big deal:** Phone interview with John Moon, February 2019.

226 **Laypeople who had no idea:** Diary/notes from the Papers of Nancy L. Caroline.

226 **"the most skilled:** Ibid.

227 **She sat on the curb:** Ibid.

228 **"Go ahead and intubate:** Ibid.

228 **His hands were trembling:** Ibid.

228 **"Um . . . you kinda:** Ibid.
229 **George took it in stride:** Ibid.
229 ***Let's get the hell outta here*****:** Ibid.
230 **"What is this?":** Ibid.
230 **"Who did this?":** Ibid.
231 **But all along:** Ibid.
231 **That's why she opened doors:** Ibid.
232 **"I intubated:** Ibid.

CHAPTER THIRTY-FIVE

234 **when they were awarded the DOT:** Page, *The Paramedics*, 35.
234 **there was no way the city could disown:** Phone interview with John Moon, February 2019.
234 **In the span of just a few months:** Ibid.
234 **John was almost afraid to touch it:** Phone interview with John Moon, March 2021.
235 **"how many more lives:** "Pete's Program: Civilians to Man New Ambulances," *Pittsburgh Post-Gazette*, May 2, 1975, 6.
235 **to saddle them with the Inebriate Program:** "City Phasing in Drunk Program," *Pittsburgh Post-Gazette*, January 16, 1975, 5.
236 **A whopping $3 million:** "City's 'Super Ambulances' Ready for Road, but Await Plan," *Pittsburgh Press*, August 18, 1975, 2.
236 **In a surprise move:** Ibid.
236 **Instead, the mayor partnered:** Ibid.
236 **$35,000 units:** "Pete's Program: Civilians to Man New Ambulances."
236 **Unfortunately, when they crept close:** Phone interview with John Moon, November 2018.
236 **"I need, fairly urgently:** Letter from Nancy Caroline to Peter Safar, from the Papers of Nancy L. Caroline,1905–2007.
237 **they'd already begun staffing:** Phone interview with John Moon, May 2021.
237 **Community College of Allegheny County:** Ibid.
237 **When they came:** Ibid.
237 **"What do you want me to do?":** Ibid.
237 **They took the newer:** Ibid.
238 **Glenn Cannon, whom Flaherty tapped:** "Pete's Program: Civilians to Man New Ambulances."
238 **But it was beyond galling:** Phone interview with John Moon, May 2021.

238 **"During those years:** "Emergency!," *Pittsburgh Magazine* (April 1977): 86.

238 **Cannon expressed indifference:** Letter from Nancy Caroline to Peter Safar, from the Papers of Nancy L. Caroline.

238 **And so Nancy was offered the job:** Ibid.

238 **"considerable, uneasy thought,":** Ibid.

239 **"laudable":** Letter from Peter Safar to Nancy Caroline, from the Papers of Nancy L. Caroline.

CHAPTER THIRTY-SIX

240 **It happened in March:** Obituary for Manuel Soto Curiel, *Kansas City Star*, March 16, 1975, 8.

240 **Manny's demons rose:** Diary/notes from the Papers of Nancy L. Caroline, 1905–2007.

240 **A typical night:** Letter from Nancy Caroline to Jonathan Gill, from the Papers of Nancy L. Caroline.

240 **"maddening,":** Letter from Jonathan Gill to Nancy Caroline, from the Papers of Nancy L. Caroline.

240 **She was aware of Nancy:** Letter from Claudia Curiel to Nancy Caroline, March 1975, from the Papers of Nancy L. Caroline.

240 **"reaching for somebody.":** Ibid.

241 **Alice in Wonderland:** Letter from Nancy Caroline to Jonathan Gill, from the Papers of Nancy L. Caroline.

241 **Manny ingested ammonia:** Ibid.

241 **"one day some defense:** Ibid.

241 **"massive dose of human:** Letter from Nancy Caroline to Peter Safar, from the Papers of Nancy L. Caroline.

241 **Indeed, there was nothing:** Ibid.

242 **"There are thirty human beings:** Ibid.

CHAPTER THIRTY-SEVEN

243 **Quietly shouldering a burden:** Phone interview with John Moon, November 2021.

244 **"It happened like this:** Diary/notes from the Papers of Nancy L. Caroline.

244 **"Put him in Western Psych:** Ibid.

244 **"He's a karate:** Ibid.

245 **John sighed and peered:** Phone interview with John Moon, February 2019.

245 **But they were angry:** Phone interview with Bill Raynovich, October 2020.

245 **"You've got a jewel:** Ibid.

245 **"Is that what you're going to do?":** Phone interview with John Moon, January 2021.

245 **Nancy was determined:** Letter from Nancy Caroline to Peter Safar, from the Papers of Nancy L. Caroline.

246 **"You can't give up:** Phone interview with John Moon, January 2021.

246 **"One thing about municipal:** Phone interview with John Moon, January 2021.

246 **"anxious to avoid:** "Emergency!," 86.

246 **If they didn't, she had:** Letter from Nancy Caroline to Peter Safar, from the Papers of Nancy L. Caroline.

246 **"blackmail":** Letter from Peter Safar to Nancy Caroline, from the Papers of Nancy L. Caroline.

247 **The organization, she wrote:** "Memorandum of Intent," from Freedom House Board to Mayor Pete Flaherty, from the Papers of Nancy L. Caroline.

247 **"the city will arrange:** Ibid.

247 **except the last:** Letter from Mayor Pete Flaherty to Freedom House, from the Papers of Nancy L. Caroline.

CHAPTER THIRTY-EIGHT

248 **"you'll always be:** Letter from Robert Zepfel to Nancy Caroline, October 1975, from the Papers of Nancy L. Caroline, 1905–2007, Schlesinger Library, Radcliffe Institute, Harvard University.

248 **"though we will be disbanded:** Letter from Robert Zepfel to Peter Safar, October 1975, from the Papers of Nancy L. Caroline.

248 **medics kept their letter:** Phone interview with John Moon, March 2021.

248 **"All of you have reason to be proud:** Letter from Nancy Caroline to Freedom House medics upon closing, from the Papers of Nancy L. Caroline.

248 **"You have profoundly:** Ibid.

248 **"It has been a rare privilege:** Ibid.

249 **One afternoon:** "Emergency!," 86.

249 **"If you take:** Letter from Nancy Caroline to Freedom House medics.

249 **"There are pieces:** Diary/notes from the Papers of Nancy L. Caroline.

249 **"Freedom House should be:** Letter from Nancy Caroline to Freedom House.

249 **"We need someone:** Diary/notes from the Papers of Nancy L. Caroline.

249 **"This is the end:** Letter from Nancy Caroline to Freedom House medics.

249 **"But it need not be:** Ibid.

CHAPTER THIRTY-NINE

250 **On the night of:** Phone interview with John Moon, November 2018; Faulk Medical Fund archives, Heinz History Center, Pittsburgh.

250 **"This is Mr. Zepfel:** Ibid.

250 **John stared through the window:** Phone interview with John Moon, November 2018.

250 **They all did, except Raynovich:** Phone interview with Bill Raynovich, October 2020.

251 **Nancy got drunk:** Diary/notes from the Papers of Nancy L. Caroline, 1905–2007.

251 **"Eight years:** "Emergency!" *Pittsburgh Magazine* (April 1977): 86.

251 **John wondered:** Phone interview with John Moon, November 2018.

CHAPTER FORTY

252 **"Over the ensuing months,":** "Emergency!," 86.

252 **The first hint of things to come:** Mitch Brown, remarks during webinar.

252 **Cannon called back:** Ibid.

252 **"warmth":** "Super Ambulance Plan Lacks Warmth, Empathy, City Told," *Pittsburgh Press*, October 24, 1975, 3.

253 **There was no pride:** Phone interview with John Moon, June 2021.

253 **evidence of a grocery store:** "Hill House Geared to Meet Almost Anyone's Needs," *Pittsburgh Post-Gazette*, March 26, 1975, 17.

253 ***Here we go again*:** Phone interview with John Moon, June 2021.

253 **"Who's this?":** Ibid.

253 **"Oh. That's:** Ibid.

254 **They were equipped:** Ibid.

254 **When Raynovich arrived:** Phone interview with Bill Raynovich, October 2020.

254 **"a goon squad.":** Ibid.

254 **white only on the outside:** Ibid.

254 **"I became a second-class:** Phone interview with John Moon, June 2021.

255 **Darnella was the last one in:** Phone interview conducted with Darnella Wilson, August 2020.

255 **But Walt had other ideas:** Ibid.

255 **"You need a job.":** Ibid.

255 ***if I do something wrong*****:** Ibid.

256 **"What are y'all doing:** Ibid.

256 **"I don't know:** Ibid.

256 **Darnella grew up:** Ibid.

256 **Darnella was never sure:** Ibid.

257 **Darnella found her purpose:** Ibid.

257 **but it wasn't forced to keep them:** Phone interview with John Moon, June 2021.

257 **driven by racism and spite:** Phone interview with John Moon, June 2021; phone interview conducted with Darnella Wilson, August 2020; phone interview with Bill Raynovich, October 2020.

257 **forced to take yet another course:** Phone interview with John Moon, June 2021; phone interview with Darnella Wilson, August 2020.

257 **Nancy was livid:** "Emergency!"; phone interview with John Moon, June 2021.

258 **The medics hired by the city:** Phone interview with John Moon, June 2021; phone interview with Bill Raynovich, October 2020.

258 **Though hired as a paramedic:** Phone interview with John Moon, June 2021.

258 **The Hill was a place:** Ibid.

258 **armed with knives, brass knuckles:** Ibid.

259 **It happened:** Ibid.

259 **One night, Raynovich returned:** Phone interview with Bill Raynovich, October 2020.

259 **Nancy fought for the medics:** Phone interview with Bill Raynovich, October 2020; phone interview with John Moon, June 2021; letter from Ames Coney Jr. to Phil Hallen, September 1976, Faulk Medical Fund archives, Heinz History Center, Pittsburgh.

259 **"city never accepted:** Letter from Aims Coney Jr. to Phil Hallen.

259 **"personnel who transferred:** Ibid.

259 **a living hell:** Phone interview with Darnella Wilson, August 2020.

260 **it was horrible and traumatizing:** Ibid.

260 **Within that first year:** Phone interview with Bill Raynovich, October 2020; phone interview with John Moon, June 2021; "Emergency!"

260 **Ron Ragin, part of the original:** Phone interview with John Moon, June 2021; Freedom House employee rolls, from the Papers of Nancy L. Caroline, 1905–2007, Schlesinger Library, Radcliffe Institute, Harvard University.

260 **Then McCary:** Phone interview with John Moon, June 2021.

261 ***they're trying to fire me*:** Ibid.

261 **They formed study groups:** Phone interview with John Moon, February 2019.

261 **"Okay,":** Phone interview with John Moon, June 2021.

CHAPTER FORTY-ONE

262 **It felt like the old days:** Phone interview with John Moon, June 2021.

263 **"Do something!":** Ibid.

EPILOGUE

265 **A constant clack:** Diary/notes from the Papers of Nancy L. Caroline, 1905–2007, Schlesinger Library, Radcliffe Institute, Harvard University.

265 **The class she taught:** Nancy Caroline, draft of "Emergency Care in the Streets," from the Papers of Nancy L. Caroline.

265 **It sounded like a good idea:** Diary/notes from the Papers of Nancy L. Caroline.

265 **Audrey loaned her an electric space heater:** Ibid.

266 **In June she left:** Ibid.; letter from Aims Coney Jr. to Phil Hallen, September 1976, Faulk Medical Fund archives, Heinz History Center, Pittsburgh.

266 **John Bucci and John Barnett:** Freedom House employee rolls.

266 **Darnella Wilson fought through:** Phone interview with Darnella Wilson, August 2020.

266 **Raynovich was another one:** Phone interview with Bill Raynovich, October 2020.

266 **Dave Rayzer earned:** Freedom House employee rolls.

267 **Gerald Esposito, the man:** Ibid.

267 **Others left medicine:** Ibid.

267 **"I have wisely used:** Letter sent from George McCary to Nancy Caroline, May 1977, from the Papers of Nancy L. Caroline.

267 **Mitch Brown became:** "A Departing Mitchell Brown Looks Back," *University Times*, January 24, 1980, 2.

267 **"Well, you call the best:** Mitch Brown, remarks during webinar hosted by the University of Pittsburgh Graduate School of Public Health, September 2020.

267 **Phil Hallen remained:** Phone interview with Phil Hallen, March 2019.

268 **Eva once described:** Phone interview with Eva Safar, August 2020.

268 **In 1979 he stepped down:** "Careers in Anesthesiology," Safar, 246.

268 **In later years, he lamented:** Ibid., 6.

268 **He remained altruistic but admitted:** Ibid., 345.

268 **He'd resisted efforts:** Ibid., 140.

268 **Safar never asked for:** Ibid., 146–147.

268 **Annie's face was modeled after:** "Resusci Anne and L'Inconnue: The Mona Lisa of the Seine," *BBC News*, October 16, 2013.

269 **In 1977, Nancy realized:** Introduction to the Papers of Nancy L. Caroline.

269 **It wasn't an easy task:** Phone interview with Oren Wacht, March 2019.

269 **received by some with skepticism:** Ibid.

269 **On March 11, 1978:** "Terrorists! Med-Emergency!" *Jewish Chronicle of Pittsburgh*, April 26, 1979, 8.

270 **"presumably looking for terrorists:** Letter from Nancy Caroline to Peter Safar, Peter Safar Papers, 1950–2003, University of Pittsburgh archives.

270 **founded Hospice of the Upper Galilee:** "A Leader in Preparing Nonphysicians to Provide Emergency Medical Care," *Pittsburgh Post-Gazette*, December 21, 2002, 4.

270 **"Israel's Mother Teresa.":** Phone interview with Oren Wacht, March 2019; "Israel's Mother Teresa to Be Buried in Boston," *Jerusalem Post*, December 15, 2002.

270 **"peculiar bond with remote events:** Diary/notes from the Papers of Nancy L. Caroline.

271 **"the little nurse:** "Ex-Commissioner William Hunt Is Dead at 76," *Pittsburgh Post-Gazette*, July 21, 1990, 8.

271 **When the next slot:** Phone interview with John Moon, February 2021.

271 **He and Betty separated:** Phone interview with John Moon, December 2021.

272 **it got him thinking:** Phone interview with John Moon, February 2021.

272 **(in 1997 Pittsburgh would become:** "Federal Intervention in Local Policing: Pittsburgh's Experience with a Consent Decree," Office of Justice Programs, US Department of Justice, October 2006.

272 **it hit John all at once:** Phone interview with John Moon, February 2021.

273 **end a law that said:** Ibid.

273 **He created a program:** Ibid.

273 **In 2002, he successfully:** Ibid.

273 **"Mr. Moon was instrumental:** Mitch Brown, remarks during webinar.

273 **"Hell yeah.":** Phone interview with Darnella Wilson, August 2020.

274 **after he channeled the spirit of George McCary:** Phone interview with John Moon, February 2021.

DISCUSSION GUIDE FOR AMERICAN SIRENS

1. Before the development of the pioneering ambulance service called Freedom House, what were the options for a person experiencing a medical emergency? What values and ideas about city and state government might explain such limited help for citizens?

2. Who is John Moon? What aspects of his childhood were challenging and painful? In what ways was the Carrie Steele-Pitts Home helpful to him or not? What did adults seem to fail to understand about John's anger?

3. In what ways might John Moon's difficult and lonely childhood years have influenced his decisions to work as an orderly and then as a paramedic? What particular qualities and characteristics did he bring to the new, challenging work of Freedom House?

4. When John Moon first saw the Freedom House paramedics deliver an emergency patient to Montefiore, what specifics about them and their work struck him so powerfully?

5. What was the "viciously destructive policy known as urban renewal"? What population did this policy harm the most? What was its legacy for cities, neighborhoods, and those who

lived there? What systemic policies and laws were used to justify such destruction of neighborhoods and the segregation of those that replaced them? How was it all related to a service like Freedom House?

6. Who was Emily Dunning? What forces were used to try to prevent her from working in ambulance medicine despite her vastly outperforming men considered to be the country's best doctors? How did she eventually succeed?

7. What was Peter Safar like? What qualities and experience made him "the ideal person for this moment" of the evolution of Freedom House? In what important ways did he push against political and systemic discrimination of the time?

8. Peter Safar was "driven by something other than his refusal to turn away from a challenge, something far more personal." What might this have been? What might explain his vision of racial equality?

9. What was it about "street medicine" and "ambulance care" that didn't seem like "real medicine" to people? What kinds of emergencies began to change public and political opinion about the value of this new kind of treatment?

10. Why did Peter Safar want "ordinary people" to train to become paramedics for Freedom House? What did he believe was necessary to transform "life-failures to life-givers"?

11. What might it mean that "grassroots community organizing was jazz, unstructured and free"? How is it different from and possibly hampered by more rigid and regulated political and social systems?

12. Who were the various first students of Freedom House? How was each different from the others? What attributes in particular did they bring to the group and the work? What was important about the idea that "if medicine teaches you anything, it's that we all bleed red and die easy"?

13. What kinds of indignities did the students of Freedom House endure during their training? What powerful and admirable qualities did they demonstrate in the face of this treatment?

14. What was particularly powerful about the kind of work the Freedom House paramedics were doing? How did it affect them as individuals? What might it mean to be "touching a moment that felt close to grace"?

15. What powerful political, financial, and legal obstacles did Freedom House face despite its groundbreaking, elite service? How was a politician like Peter Flaherty able to communicate his racist ideas about Freedom House to the "silent majority"? What hypocritical explanations did he use to deny any support to Freedom House?

16. In what other ways did Freedom House and its dedicated workers encounter discrimination and racism? What was their relationship to the police?

17. Why did Nancy Caroline take the position of medical director for Freedom House? What unique and powerful ideas and abilities did she bring to the work? What challenge in her personal life was she struggling with at the time?

18. Why did Nancy Caroline decide she had to be "maximally obnoxious" to help rebuild Freedom House? In what ways

did she experience sexist discrimination in her work? How did it help her identify and work with the members of Freedom House?

19. What might it mean that for Nancy, "all the laughing and yelling, the talking, the shit-talking, the *yeah, but for real* talking" with those of Freedom House "sustained her"? What might she mean when she says her overall experience with Freedom House had "saved" her?

20. What many systemic and discriminatory forces explain how the profound work, success, and even jobs were largely taken from those of Freedom House when ambulance care was finally accepted and valued by larger, white society? How is it that politicians can simply break promises they have made publicly and not be held accountable?

21. What were the various and harmful effects of the shift in power dynamics and authority that put unskilled white workers in charge of the elite workers of Freedom House, most of whom were Black? In what other ways did the city, "driven by racism and spite," work to weed out those from Freedom House?

22. What experience helped John Moon reclaim a position of expertise and power in his ambulance unit? How did he continue to evolve in his work in emergency medicine? What factors contributed to his admirable success?

23. What is the legacy of Freedom House? What is particularly important to understand about it and the dedicated and compassionate people who were part of it?